STRETCHING ANATOMY

Arnold G. Nelson
Jouko Kokkonen

Illustrated by
Jason M. McAlexander

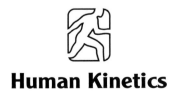

Human Kinetics

Library of Congress Cataloging-in-Publication Data

Nelson, Arnold G., 1953-
  Stretching anatomy / Arnold G. Nelson, Jouko Kokkonen.
     p. cm.
  Includes index.
  ISBN-13: 978-0-7360-5972-5 (soft cover)
  ISBN-10: 0-7360-5972-5 (soft cover)
  1. Muscles--Anatomy. 2. Stretch (Physiology) I. Kokkonen, Jouko, 1950- II. Title.
  QM151.N45 2007
  613.7'182--dc22

                                                    2006013908

ISBN-10: 0-7360-5972-5
ISBN-13: 978-0-7360-5972-5

Acquisitions Editor: Martin Barnard; **Developmental Editor:** Leigh Keylock; **Assistant Editor:** Christine Horger; **Copyeditor:** Jan Feeney; **Proofreader:** Bethany Bentley; **Graphic Designer:** Fred Starbird; **Graphic Artist:** Tara Welsch; **Cover Designer:** Keith Blomberg; **Art Manager:** Kelly Hendren; **Illustrator (cover and interior):** Jason M. McAlexander; **Printer:** United Graphics

Human Kinetics books are available at special discounts for bulk purchase. Special editions or book excerpts can also be created to specification. For details, contact the Special Sales Manager at Human Kinetics.

Printed in the United States of America   10 9 8 7 6 5

Human Kinetics
Web site: www.HumanKinetics.com

United States: Human Kinetics
P.O. Box 5076
Champaign, IL 61825-5076
800-747-4457
e-mail: humank@hkusa.com

Canada: Human Kinetics
475 Devonshire Road, Unit 100
Windsor, ON N8Y 2L5
800-465-7301 (in Canada only)
e-mail: orders@hkcanada.com

Europe: Human Kinetics
107 Bradford Road
Stanningley
Leeds LS28 6AT, United Kingdom
+44 (0)113 255 5665
e-mail: hk@hkeurope.com

Australia: Human Kinetics
57A Price Avenue
Lower Mitcham, South Australia 5062
08 8372 0999
e-mail: info@hkaustralia.com

New Zealand: Human Kinetics
Division of Sports Distributors NZ Ltd.
P.O. Box 300 226 Albany
North Shore City, Auckland
0064 9 448 1207
e-mail: info@humankinetics.co.nz

CONTENTS

INTRODUCTION

Good flexibility is known to bring positive benefits in the muscles and joints. It aids with injury prevention, helps to minimize muscle soreness, and improves efficiency in all physical activities. Increasing flexibility can also improve quality of life and functional independence. Good flexibility aids in the elasticity of the muscles and provides a wider range of motion in the joints. It provides ease in body movements and everyday activities. A simple daily task such as bending over and tying shoes is accomplished better with flexibility.

Unfortunately, flexibility is generally not a focus of people wanting to start a fitness program. In fact, many times it is minimally addressed or neglected altogether. While the benefits of regular cardiovascular and strength training exercise are well known, few people realize that flexible joints and regular stretching are also essential for optimum health and activity. Recently, many whole-body fitness and wellness programs, such as yoga and Pilates, which incorporate some flexibility training, have increased in popularity. While these programs may improve the flexibility of individual body segments, their emphasis is not specifically aimed at improving the range of motion of all of the major joints. Yoga emphasizes balance in all areas, seeks to strengthen all muscle groups equally, creates balance between the mental and physical, and encourages moderation in everything. Yoga involves holding static poses while exploring breathing, physical feelings, and emotions. The increase in flexibility comes from holding the body in the desired poses. Pilates, on the other hand, is an exercise program that encourages the use of the mind to control the muscles. It emphasizes strengthening the postural muscles that help keep the body balanced and provide support for the spine. In contrast to traditional strength training programs that involve multiple sets and repetitions of a single exercise, a Pilates workout stresses few repetitions of each exercise and emphasizes doing these movements with precise control and form. The increases in flexibility are primarily accomplished from the ballistic movements used to increase strength.

How much stretching should a person do every day? Usually, most stretching tends to be a very brief routine concentrating on the muscle groups of the lower body. The total time spent in a stretching routine hardly ever exceeds 5 minutes; people tend to stretch a particular muscle group for no more than 15 seconds. Additionally, the stretching usually occurs at the start of the exercise session. Even in sport training, stretching is given minor importance in the overall training programs. An athlete might spend just a little more time stretching than the average person. This is usually because it is part of a warm-up routine. After the workout, however, most athletes are either too tired to do any stretching or simply do not take the time to do it. To be the most effective, however, stretching should be performed both during warm-up before a workout routine and as part of a cool-down after the workout.

For any person, whether an athlete or not, a regular stretching routine can bring some interesting benefits. Research studies on hamstring injuries have shown that those people with the lowest flexibility have the greatest chance of injury. Interestingly, the type of increased flexibility needed for reducing injury did not come from doing stretching exercises right before the activity. Rather, the increased flexibility required for fewer injuries came only from doing weeks of stretch training. Additional research has shown that regular, intense stretching for a minimum of 10 minutes will bring some major beneficial changes in the neuromuscular–tendon units. Increased strength and endurance gains have been reported as well as improved flexibility and mobility.

Types of Stretching

In general, any movement that requires moving a body part to the point at which there is an increase in the movement of a joint can be called a stretching exercise. Stretching can be done either actively or passively. Active stretching occurs when the person doing the stretch is the one holding the body part in the stretched position. Passive stretching occurs when someone else moves the person to the stretch position and then holds the person in the position for a set time. The four major types of stretches are static, proprioceptive neuromuscular facilitation (PNF), ballistic, and dynamic. The static stretch is used most often. In static stretching, one stretches a particular muscle or group of muscles by slowly moving the body part into position and then holding the stretch for a set time. Since the static stretch begins with a relaxed muscle and then applies the stretch slowly, static stretching does not activate the stretch reflex (the knee jerk seen when the tendon is tapped with a mallet). Activation of the stretch reflex causes the stretched muscle to contract instead of elongate. This contraction of the muscle is directly opposite of the intent of the exercise. PNF stretching refers to a stretching technique in which a fully contracted muscle is stretched by moving a limb through the joint's range of motion. After moving through the complete range of motion, the muscle is relaxed and rested before resuming the procedure. The combination of muscle contraction and stretching serves to relax the muscles used to maintain muscle tone. This relaxation allows for increased flexibility by "quieting" the internal forces in both the muscles that assist and the ones that oppose the movement of the joint in the desired direction. Ballistic stretching uses muscle contractions to force muscle elongation through bobbing movements where there is no pause at any point in the movement. Although the bobbing movement quickly elongates the muscle with each repetition, the bobbing also activates the stretch reflex (or knee jerk) response. Since the stretch reflex stimulates the muscle groups to contract after the stretch is finished, ballistic stretching is usually discouraged. Dynamic stretching refers to the stretching that occurs while performing sport-specific movements. Dynamic stretching is similar to ballistic stretching in that both use fast body movements to cause muscle stretch, but dynamic stretching does not employ bouncing or bobbing. Additionally, dynamic stretching uses only the muscle actions specific to a sport. Practically speaking, dynamic stretching is similar to performing a sport-specific warm-up (that is, performing the movements required for the activity but at a lower intensity).

Benefits of Stretching

The following are several chronic training benefits gained from using a regular stretching program:

- Improved flexibility, stamina (muscular endurance), and muscular strength. The degree of benefit depends on how much stress is put on the muscle. Medium or heavy stretches are recommended. You can do this by building up to doing long stretches of high intensity (see the next section for a detailed explanation of light, medium, and heavy stretching).
- Reduced muscle soreness, aches, and pains. Use only very light stretches if muscle soreness prevails.
- Improved flexibility with the use of static or PNF stretches. Medium or heavy stretches are recommended.
- Good muscular and joint mobility.
- More efficient muscular movements and fluidity of motion.

- Greater ability to exert maximum force through a wider range of motion.
- Prevention of some lower back problems.
- Improved appearance and self-image.
- Improved body alignment and posture.
- Better warm-up and cool-down in an exercise session.

General Recommendations

- Try to include all the major muscle groups in any stretching program.
- Do at least two different stretches for each joint movement.
- Before any physical activity, use light stretches as part of the warm-up.
- After an exercise routine, cool down with medium-intensity stretches.
- If muscles are sore after exercising, use only light stretches two or three times with a 5- to 10-second hold for each stretch performed.
- If muscle soreness persists for several days, continue using light stretches two or three times with a 5- to 10-second hold for each stretch performed.
- The majority of the stretches should be static.

Stretching Programs

The following programs can be prescribed for anyone who is interested in improving flexibility, strength, and strength endurance. To make changes to any of these areas, you need to be involved in a regular stretching program, preferably as a daily routine or as close to that as possible. Changes will not come in a day or two but rather after a dedicated effort of several weeks. You can incorporate these programs with or without any other kind of exercise routine. According to the latest research, heavy stretching, even without any other exercise activity, can bring about changes in flexibility, strength, and muscular endurance.

As in any other exercise program, progression is an integral part of a successful stretching program. The stretching progression should be gradual, going from a lighter load with less time spent on each stretch to a heavier load with more time spent on each stretch. For the programs outlined in this introduction, you should begin with the initial program, or level I, and then progress through to level V. However, you may customize this program according to your current level of experience and flexibility. Generally, working through each level at the recommended speed will result in meaningful and consistent workouts. After such workouts, you will find improved flexibility in the muscles you worked as well as the satisfaction of having done something beneficial.

Intensity is always a critical factor when you want changes and improvements to come from an exercise program. In a stretching routine, intensity is controlled by the amount of pain associated with the stretch. Using a pain scale from 0 to 10, initial pain is light (scale of 1 to 3) and usually dissipates as the time of stretching is extended. Light stretching occurs when you stretch a particular muscle group only to a point where you feel the stretch with an associated light pain. Moderate stretching (scale of 4 to 6) occurs when you start to feel increased, or "medium," pain in the muscle you're stretching. In heavy stretching (scale of 7 to 10), you will initially experience a moderate to heavy pain at the start of the stretch, but this pain slowly dissipates as stretching continues. Research studies have shown that heavier stretches rather than lighter stretches provide greater improvements in flexibility and strength. Thus, you are the key to your own success, and how well you are able to monitor stretch intensity and tolerate the pain level determines how quick and large the improvements will be.

Because of the complexity of muscle attachments, many stretching exercises simultaneously affect a variety of muscle groups in the body and stretch the muscle groups around multiple joints. Thus, a small change in body position can change the nature of a stretch on any particular muscle. To get the maximal stretching benefit in any muscle, it is helpful to know joint movements that each muscle can do. Putting the joint through the full range of each motion allows for maximal stretching.

You can customize the exercises in this book, which will allow for numerous stretch combinations. Also, this book illustrates only a portion of the available stretches. You are encouraged to experiment with these stretches by following the explanations provided. Information is also provided to enable you to explore a variety of positions in order to stretch the muscle by slightly altering the angles and directions of the various body positions. Thus, you can adapt the stretching exercises to fit your individual needs and desires. For example, if you have soreness in only one of the muscles or just a part of the muscle, you can adapt each exercise to stretch that particular muscle. If the explained stretch or particular body position does not stretch a particular muscle as much as you want it to, then experiment by slightly altering the position. Keep making alterations in the position until you reach the desired level of stretch (using a pain scale rating).

In the programs that appear in the following section, specific instructions are given relating to the time to hold the stretch and time to rest between each stretch, as well as the number of repetitions you should do. You should follow these instructions in order to get the benefits described. For example, if the instructions indicate that you should hold a stretch position for 10 seconds, time (or count out) the stretch to ensure that you hold it for the recommended time. Also, you should incorporate only two to four heavier stretching days in each week and have a lighter stretching day in between each of the heavier stretching days.

Finally, for any stretch involving sitting or lying down, you should do the stretch with a cushion underneath you, such as a carpet or athletic mat. Cushioning makes the exercises more comfortable to perform. However, the cushioning should be firm. Too soft of a cushion will reduce the effectiveness of the stretches.

RECOMMENDED PROGRAMS

The following programs are specific stretching recommendations and are based on your initial flexibility. In addition to following the programs listed, you should follow the general recommendations listed previously. Stay on each level for two to four weeks before going to the next level.

Level I

- Hold the stretching position for 5 to 10 seconds.
- Rest for 5 to 10 seconds between each stretch.
- Repeat each stretch two times.
- Use an intensity level on the scale from 1 to 3, with light pain.
- Duration is 15 to 20 minutes each session.
- Stretch two or three times per week.

Level II

- Hold the stretching position for 10 to 15 seconds.
- Rest for 10 to 15 seconds between each stretch.
- Repeat each stretch three times.
- Use an intensity level on the scale from 2 to 4, with light to moderate pain, one or two times per week.
- Use an intensity level on the scale from 1 to 2, one or two times per week.
- Duration is 20 to 30 minutes each session.
- Stretch three or four times per week.

Level III

- Hold the stretching position for 15 to 20 seconds.
- Rest for 15 to 20 seconds between each stretch.
- Repeat each stretch four times.
- Use an intensity level on the scale from 4 to 6, with moderate pain, two or three times per week.
- Use an intensity level on the scale from 1 to 4, two or three times per week.
- Duration is 30 to 40 minutes each session.
- Stretch four or five times per week.

Level IV

- Hold the stretching position for 20 to 25 seconds.
- Rest for 20 to 25 seconds between each stretch.
- Repeat each stretch five times.
- Use an intensity level on the scale from 6 to 8, with moderate to heavy pain, two or three times per week.
- Use an intensity level on the scale from 1 to 6, two or three times per week.
- Duration is 40 to 50 minutes each session.
- Stretch four or five times per week.

Level V

- Hold the stretching position for 25 to 30 seconds.
- Rest for 25 to 30 seconds between each stretch.
- Repeat each stretch five or six times.
- Use an intensity level on the scale from 8 to 10, with heavy pain, two or three times per week.
- Use an intensity level on the scale from 1 to 8, two or three times per week.
- Duration is 50 to 60 minutes each session.
- Stretch four or five times per week.

In the neck, the muscles are located in two triangular regions called the anterior and posterior triangles. The borders of the anterior triangle are the mandible (jawbone), the sternum (breast bone), and the sternocleidomastoid muscle. The major anterior muscles are the sternocleidomastoid and scalene. The borders of the posterior triangle are the clavicle (collarbone), sternocleidomastoid muscle, and trapezius muscle. The major posterior muscles are the trapezius, longissimus capitis, semispinalis capitis, and splenius capitis. The muscles in the neck are involved primarily in supporting or moving the head. The head movements are flexion (head tilted forward), extension (head tilted backward), lateral flexion and extension (head up and back sideward), and rotation. Since the muscles in the neck come in right and left pairings, all of the neck muscles are involved with lateral flexion and extension. For example, the right sternocleidomastoid helps perform right lateral flexion, and the left sternocleidomastoid helps perform right lateral extension. Illustrations showing the muscles and movements as well as a chart showing which muscles do a specific movement are located at the end of the chapter (pages 6-7).

When people think about doing stretching exercises, they seldom consider the neck muscles. Neck flexibility probably does not cross your mind until you discover that you have a stiff neck. A stiff neck is commonly associated with sleeping in a strange position (such as on a long flight), but a stiff neck can result from almost any type of physical activity. This is especially true for any activity where the head must be held in a constant stable position. Thus, a stiff neck can also have a negative effect in sports where head position is important (such as golf) or where rapid head movements are important for tracking the flight of an object (such as in racket sports). Poor neck flexibility usually results from holding the head in the same position for long periods. In addition, a fatigued neck muscle can stiffen up after exercise. The following exercises can help keep the neck from stiffening up after exercise, unusual postures, or awkward sleep positions.

Since all of the major muscles in the neck are involved in neck rotation, it is fairly easy to stretch the neck muscles. The first consideration when choosing a particular neck stretch should be whether greater stiffness occurs with flexion or extension. Therefore, the first two exercise groups are concerned with these specific actions. Once you achieve greater flexibility in either pure flexion or pure extension, then you can add a stretch that includes lateral movement. In other words, to increase the flexibility of the neck extensors, start with the neck extensor stretch and then, as flexibility increases, add the neck extensor and rotation stretch.

Remember that overstretching (very hard stretching) causes more harm than good. Sometimes a muscle becomes stiff from overstretching. Stretching can reduce muscle tone, and when tone is reduced, the body compensates by making the muscle even tighter. For each progression, start with the position that is the least stiff and progress only when, after several days of stretching, you notice a consistent lack of stiffness during the exercise. This means that you should stretch both the agonist muscles (the muscles that cause a movement) and antagonist muscles (the muscles that oppose a movement or do the opposite movement). Also, remember that although you may have greater stiffness in one direction (right versus left), you need to stretch both sides so that you maintain proper muscle balance.

Neck Extensor Stretch

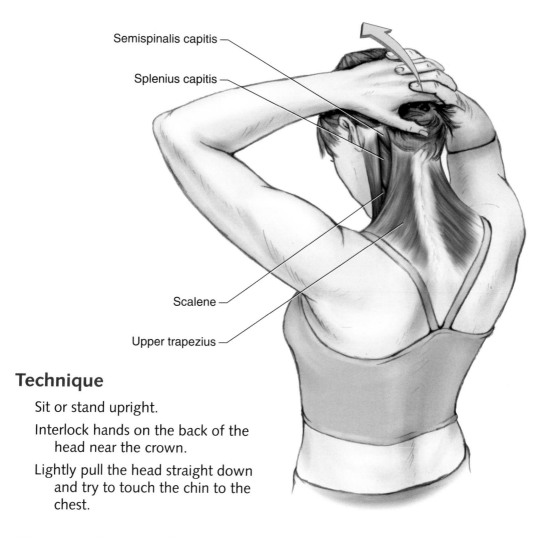

Semispinalis capitis

Splenius capitis

Scalene

Upper trapezius

Technique

Sit or stand upright.

Interlock hands on the back of the head near the crown.

Lightly pull the head straight down and try to touch the chin to the chest.

Muscles Stretched

Most-stretched muscle: Upper trapezius.

Lesser-stretched muscles: Longissimus capitis, semispinalis capitis, splenius capitis, scalene.

Commentary

You can do this stretch either while sitting or while standing. A greater stretch is applied when seated. Standing reduces the ability to stretch because reflexes come into play to prevent a loss of balance. During the stretch, make sure not to reduce the stretch by hunching up the shoulders. Also, keep the neck as straight as possible (no curving). Try to touch the chin to the lowest possible point on the chest.

Neck Extensor and Rotation Stretch

When the neck extensors become flexible, progress from stretching the right and left sides simultaneously to stretching the opposite sides individually. To do this, follow this procedure:

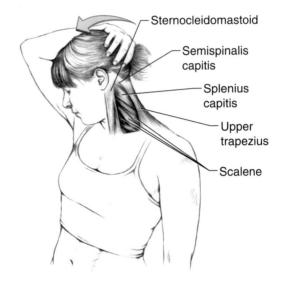

Sternocleidomastoid

Semispinalis capitis

Splenius capitis

Upper trapezius

Scalene

Technique

Sit or stand upright.

Place the right hand on the back of the head near the crown.

Pull the head down toward the right and try to touch the chin as close as possible to the right shoulder.

Muscles Stretched

Most-stretched muscles: Left upper trapezius, left sternocleidomastoid.

Lesser-stretched muscles: Left longissimus capitis, left semispinalis capitis, left splenius capitis, left scalene.

Neck Flexor Stretch

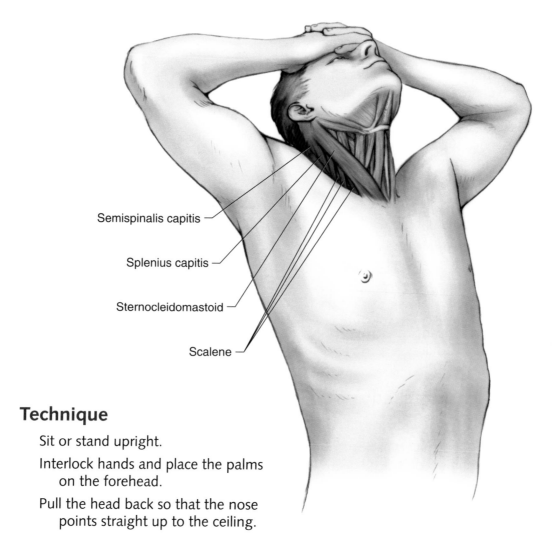

Semispinalis capitis —

Splenius capitis —

Sternocleidomastoid —

Scalene —

Technique

Sit or stand upright.

Interlock hands and place the palms on the forehead.

Pull the head back so that the nose points straight up to the ceiling.

Muscles Stretched

Most-stretched muscle: Sternocleidomastoid.

Lesser-stretched muscles: Longissimus capitis, semispinalis capitis, splenius capitis, scalene.

Commentary

You can do this stretch either while sitting or while standing. A greater stretch is applied when seated. Standing reduces the ability to stretch because reflexes come into play to prevent a loss of balance. During the stretch, make sure not to reduce the stretch by hunching up the shoulders. Also, try to point the chin as far back as possible.

Neck Flexor and Rotation Stretch

When the neck flexors become flexible, progress from stretching the right and left sides simultaneously to stretching the opposite sides individually. To do this, follow this procedure:

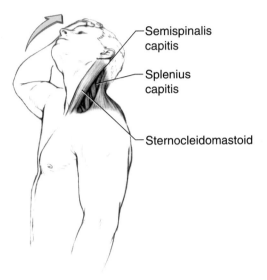

Semispinalis capitis

Splenius capitis

Sternocleidomastoid

Technique

Stand or sit upright.

Place right hand on the forehead.

Pull the head back and toward the right so that the head points toward the shoulder.

Keep the head straight; do not lay the head down to either side.

Muscles Stretched

Most-stretched muscle: Left sternocleidomastoid.

Lesser-stretched muscles: Left longissimus capitis, left semispinalis capitis, left splenius capitis.

Neck Muscle Movements

The stretches in this chapter are excellent overall stretches; however, not all of these stretches may be completely suited to each person's needs. The muscles involved in the various neck movements appear in the following table. To stretch specific muscles, the stretch must involve one or more movements in the opposite direction of the desired muscle's movements. For example, if you want to stretch the left scalene, you could extend the head both backward and laterally to the right. When a muscle has a high level of stiffness, you should use fewer simultaneous opposite movements (you would stretch a very tight right scalene by initially doing just left lateral extension). As a muscle becomes loose, you can incorporate more simultaneous opposite movements.

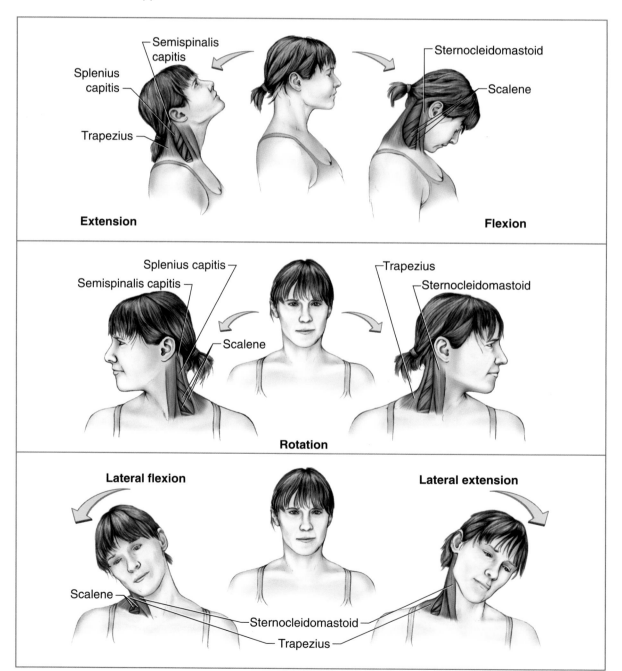

Muscle	Flexion	Extension	Rotation	Lateral flexion	Lateral extension
Longissimus capitis		✔	✔	✔	✔
Scalene	✔		✔	✔	
Semispinalis capitis		✔	✔	✔	✔
Splenius capitis		✔	✔	✔	✔
Sternocleidomastoid	✔		✔	✔	✔
Trapezius		✔	✔	✔	✔

There are five major pairs of movements at the shoulder: flexion and extension, abduction and adduction, external and internal rotation, retraction and protraction, and elevation and depression. Illustrations showing these movements as well as a chart showing which muscles do specific movements are located at the end of the chapter (pages 21-23). The bones of the shoulder joint consist of the humerus (upper arm bone), scapula (shoulder blade), and clavicle (collarbone). The scapula and clavicle essentially "float" on top of the rib cage. Therefore, a major function of many upper-back and chest muscles is to attach the scapula (in the upper back) and clavicle (in the upper chest) to the rib cage and spine. This provides a stable platform for arm and shoulder movements. Of the five movement pairs mentioned here, retraction and protraction and elevation and depression are usually classified as stabilization actions. The majority of the muscles involved in moving and stabilizing the shoulder bones are located posterior. The scapula is a much larger bone than the clavicle and has room for more muscles to attach. The posterior muscles are infraspinatus, latissimus dorsi, levator scapulae, rhomboids, subclavius, subscapularis, supraspinatus, teres major, teres minor, and trapezius (attached to the upper posterior rib cage, vertebrae [spine], and scapulae), as well as the deltoid and triceps brachii (attached to the scapulae and humerus). The anterior muscles are the pectoralis major (attached to the clavicle anterior rib cage and humerus), the pectoralis minor, and serratus anterior (attached to the anterior rib cage and anterior scapulae as well as the biceps brachii, coracobrachialis, and deltoid (attached to the anterior scapulae and humerus).

Common complaints associated with the musculature of the shoulders and upper back and chest are tight muscles and muscle spasms in the neck (middle and upper trapezius), shoulder (trapezius, deltoid, supraspinatus), and upper-back muscles (rhomboids and levator scapulae). Interestingly, the tightness felt in these muscles is usually a result of initial tightness in their antagonist muscles. In other words, tight muscles in the upper chest caused the tightness felt in the upper back. Tight chest muscles (that is, the pectoralis major) cause a constant low-level stretch on the muscles of the upper back. Eventually, this low-level stretch elongates the ligaments and tendons associated with the upper-back muscles. Once these ligaments and tendons become elongated, the tone in their associated muscles falls dramatically. To reclaim the lost tone, the muscles must increase their force of contraction. Increased force in turn causes more stretch of the ligaments and tendons, and increased muscle contraction must compensate for that. Hence, a vicious cycle commences. The best way to prevent or stop this cycle is to stretch the anterior shoulder and chest muscles. As these muscles increase in flexibility, the tightness of the posterior muscles will also be reduced. Also, immediately after stretching, the strength of the muscles is diminished. It is also a good idea to stretch the opposing muscles just before and immediately after working any group of muscles. If this is done three or more times a week, the muscles will actually increase in flexibility and gain strength. Stretching will also reduce the frequency of tightness for any group of muscles.

Many of the instructions and illustrations in this chapter are given for the left or right side of the body. Similar but opposite procedures would be used for the opposite (not pictured) side of the body.

Shoulder Flexor Stretch

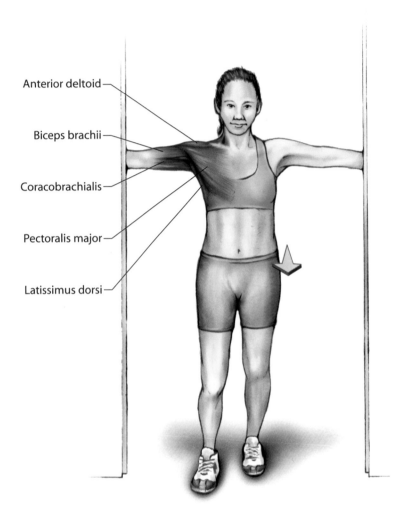

Anterior deltoid

Biceps brachii

Coracobrachialis

Pectoralis major

Latissimus dorsi

Technique

Stand upright while facing a doorway or corner.

Place feet shoulder-width apart with one foot slightly in front of the other.

With straight arms, raise your arms to shoulder level and place the palms on the walls or doorframe with the thumbs on top.

Lean the entire body forward.

Muscles Stretched

Most-stretched muscles: Pectoralis major, anterior deltoid, coracobrachialis, biceps brachii.

Lesser-stretched muscles: Infraspinatus, latissimus dorsi, subclavius, lower trapezius.

Commentary

To get the maximum benefit during the stretch, keep the elbows locked and the spine straight. The greater the forward lean, the better the stretch. Forward lean is controlled by how far the lead foot is in front of the chest at the start position. Hence, place the foot forward only enough to maintain balance. It is possible to do the neck extensor stretch simultaneously with the shoulder flexor stretch. However, without having the hands pushing down on the head, the neck extensor stretch will be of a lower intensity than if it were done by itself.

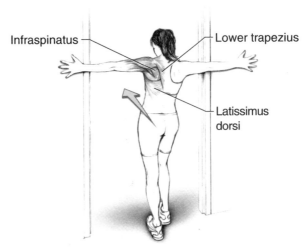

Infraspinatus

Lower trapezius

Latissimus dorsi

VARIATION

Shoulder Flexor and Depressor Stretch

Elevating the arms will stretch more muscles.

Technique

- Stand upright while facing a doorway or corner.
- Place feet shoulder-width apart with one foot slightly in front of the other.
- With straight arms, raise arms high above the head, and place the palms on the walls or doorframe.
- Lean the entire body forward.

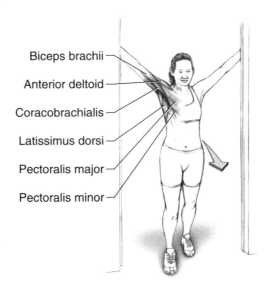

Biceps brachii

Anterior deltoid

Coracobrachialis

Latissimus dorsi

Pectoralis major

Pectoralis minor

Muscles Stretched

Most-stretched muscles: Pectoralis major, anterior deltoid, coracobrachialis, biceps brachii, pectoralis minor.

Lesser-stretched muscles: Latissimus dorsi, lower trapezius, subclavius.

Shoulder Extensor, Adductor, and Retractor Stretch

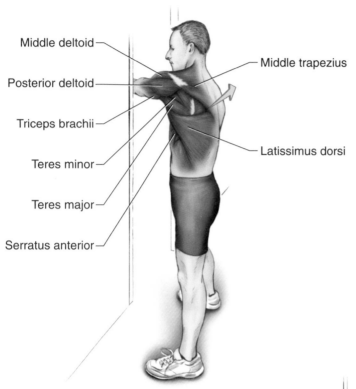

Middle deltoid

Posterior deltoid

Triceps brachii

Teres minor

Teres major

Serratus anterior

Middle trapezius

Latissimus dorsi

Technique

Stand upright inside a doorway while facing a doorjamb with the doorjamb in line with the right shoulder.

Place feet shoulder-width apart with the toes pointing straight forward.

Bring the left arm across the body toward the right shoulder.

Pointing the thumb down, grab hold of the doorjamb at shoulder level.

Rotate the trunk inward until you feel a stretch in the posterior left shoulder.

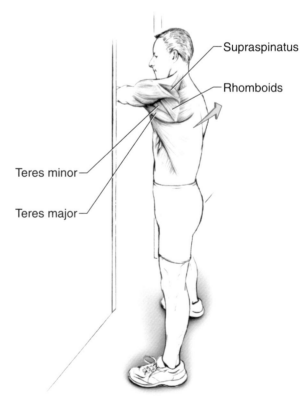

Supraspinatus

Rhomboids

Teres minor

Teres major

Muscles Stretched

Most-stretched muscles: Left posterior and middle deltoid, left latissimus dorsi, left triceps brachii, left middle trapezius, left rhomboids.

Lesser-stretched muscles: Left teres major, left teres minor, left supraspinatus, left serratus anterior.

Commentary

To get the maximum benefit of this stretch, you should keep the elbow locked. Over time, as the muscles become more flexible, to keep the elbow locked you will need to grasp the doorframe above the level of the shoulder. Raising the height of the hand does not diminish the major benefits of this stretch. However, as the hand gets higher above shoulder level, the stretch on the rhomboids decreases while the stretch on the serratus anterior increases.

Shoulder Adductor, Protractor, and Elevator Stretch

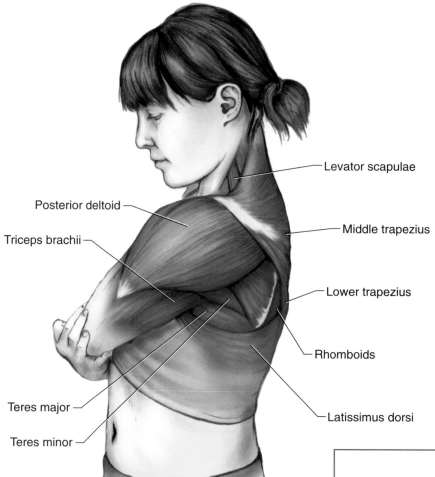

Levator scapulae

Posterior deltoid

Triceps brachii

Middle trapezius

Lower trapezius

Rhomboids

Teres major

Teres minor

Latissimus dorsi

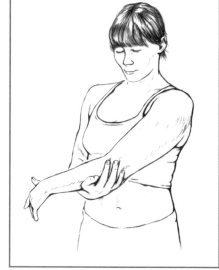

Technique

Stand upright with the feet shoulder-width apart.

Bring the left arm across the front of the body, with the left hand near the right hip.

With the right hand, grab hold of the left elbow.

With the right hand, try to pull the left elbow down and around the right side of the body.

Muscles Stretched

Most-stretched muscles: Left posterior deltoid, left latissimus dorsi, left triceps brachii, left lower middle trapezius.

Lesser-stretched muscles: Left teres major, left teres minor, left supraspinatus, left levator scapulae, left rhomboids.

Commentary

To maximize the stretch, do not raise the shoulder or bend at the waist. If it is not possible to bring the hand toward the hip, try to come as close as possible. As long as the arm is below the shoulders, the stretch will be effective for the stated muscles.

VARIATION

Shoulder Adductor, Elevator, and Protractor Stretch

Bringing the arm above the shoulder changes the emphasis of the stretch to the elevators and protractors.

Technique

- Stand upright with the feet shoulder-width apart.
- Raise the left hand high above the head, and bring the left arm up against the left side of the head.
- With the right hand, grab hold of the left elbow.
- With the right hand, try to pull the left elbow behind the head, past the left ear.

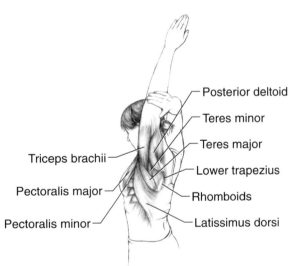

Triceps brachii — Posterior deltoid — Teres minor — Teres major — Lower trapezius — Pectoralis major — Rhomboids — Pectoralis minor — Latissimus dorsi

Muscles Stretched

Most-stretched muscles: Left posterior deltoid, left latissimus dorsi, left triceps brachii, left lower trapezius, left serratus anterior.

Lesser-stretched muscles: Left teres major, left teres minor, left supraspinatus, left rhomboids, left pectoralis minor.

One-Arm Shoulder Flexor Stretch

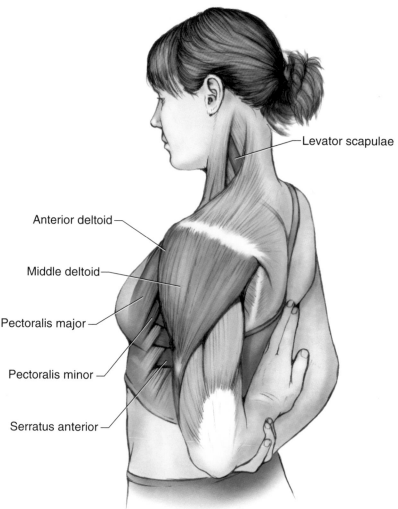

Levator scapulae

Anterior deltoid

Middle deltoid

Pectoralis major

Pectoralis minor

Serratus anterior

Technique

Stand (or sit on a backless chair) upright with the left arm behind the back and the elbow bent at about 90 degrees.

Place feet shoulder-width apart with the toes pointing forward.

Grasp the left elbow with the right hand.

Pull the left arm across the back and up toward the right shoulder.

Muscles Stretched

Most-stretched muscles: Left pectoralis major, left anterior deltoid, and middle deltoid.

Lesser-stretched muscles: Left levator scapulae, left pectoralis minor, left supraspinatus, left serratus anterior, left coracobrachialis.

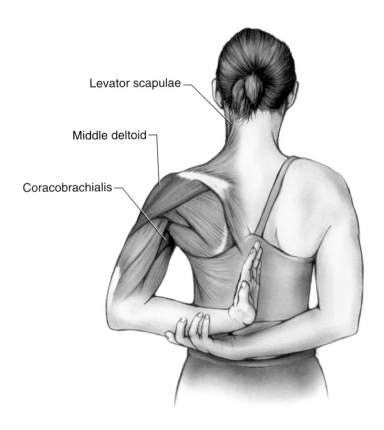

Levator scapulae

Middle deltoid

Coracobrachialis

Commentary

If you cannot reach the elbow, then grasp the wrist. When pulling on the wrist, it is easy to pull the arm across the back, but remember that the best effect comes only from pulling upward as well as across. Also, keep the elbow locked at a near-90-degree angle. Changing the alignment of the back will also influence the magnitude of the stretch. If you cannot keep the back straight, arching the back is preferable to bending at the waist. Just be careful; it is easy to lose balance when doing this stretch while both arching the back and standing up.

Shoulder Adductor and Extensor Stretch

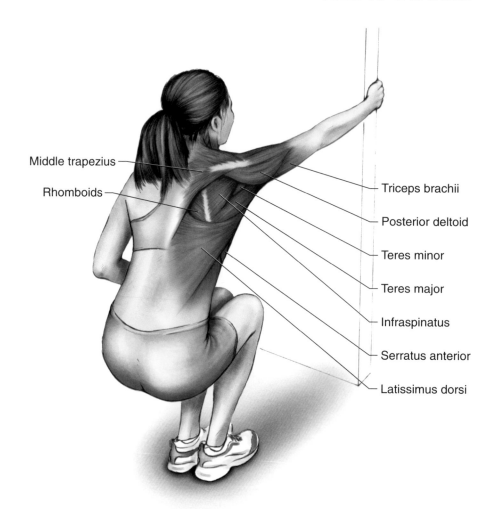

Middle trapezius

Rhomboids

Triceps brachii

Posterior deltoid

Teres minor

Teres major

Infraspinatus

Serratus anterior

Latissimus dorsi

Technique

Stand in a squatting position while facing a doorway with the right shoulder lined up with the left side of the doorjamb.

Stick the right arm through the doorway. Grab the inside of the doorjamb at shoulder level with the right hand.

While keeping the right arm straight and the feet firmly planted, lower the buttocks toward the floor.

Muscles Stretched

Most-stretched muscles: Right posterior deltoid, right middle trapezius, right triceps brachii, right teres major, right rhomboids, right infraspinatus.

Lesser-stretched muscles: Right latissimus dorsi, right teres minor, right supraspinatus, right serratus anterior.

Commentary

A lower squat yields a greater stretch, but be careful not to squat so low that you feel pain in the legs or knees. To reduce strain on the knees, change where you grab the doorjamb. Changing the position of the grasp, however, influences the amount of stretch placed on the various muscles (see variation). Regardless of where you grasp, keep the back straight or arched. Do not bend forward at the waist. To get an even greater stretch, inwardly rotate the trunk.

VARIATION

Shoulder Adductor and Extensor Stretch Variation

Changing the hand position on the doorjamb changes the muscles that you stretch.

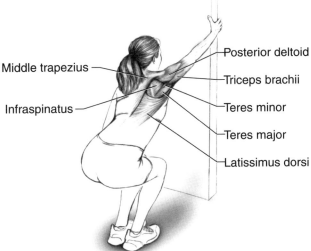

Middle trapezius

Infraspinatus

Posterior deltoid

Triceps brachii

Teres minor

Teres major

Latissimus dorsi

Technique

Stand in a squatting position while facing a doorway; line up the right shoulder with the left side of the doorjamb.

Stick the right arm through the doorway. With the right hand, grab the inside of the doorjamb above head level.

While keeping the right arm straight and the feet firmly planted, lower the buttocks toward the floor.

Muscles Stretched

Most-stretched muscles: Right posterior deltoid, right latissimus dorsi, right triceps brachii, right teres major, right infraspinatus.

Lesser-stretched muscles: Right teres minor, right supraspinatus, right middle trapezius.

Seated Shoulder Flexor Depressor Retractor Stretch

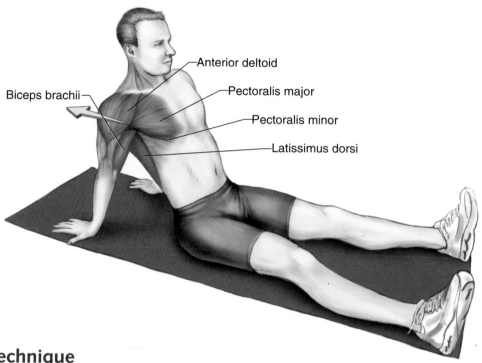

Anterior deltoid

Pectoralis major

Pectoralis minor

Latissimus dorsi

Biceps brachii

Technique

Sit on the floor with the legs straight.

While keeping the arms straight, place the palms (with the fingers pointed backward) on the floor about one foot (30 cm) behind the hips.

While keeping the arms straight, lean backward toward the floor.

Muscles Stretched

Most-stretched muscles: Pectoralis major, anterior deltoid, coracobrachialis, biceps brachii, pectoralis minor.

Lesser-stretched muscles: Latissimus dorsi, lower trapezius, subclavius, rhomboids.

Commentary

To maximize the stretch, keep the arms straight. If it is difficult to refrain from bending the arms, place the hands closer to the hips. Moving the hands farther from the hips can increase the stretch. To keep the body from sliding along the floor, you may need to brace the soles of the feet against a wall. Sitting on a mat with the hands placed on a hard surface will increase the stretch as well as add comfort.

Shoulder, Back, and Chest Muscle Movements

The stretches in this chapter are excellent overall stretches; however, not all of these stretches may be completely suited to each person's needs. The muscles involved in the various shoulder and upper chest and back movements appear in the following table. To stretch specific muscles, the stretch must involve one or more movements in the opposite direction of the desired muscle's movements. For example, if you want to stretch the serratus anterior, you could perform a movement that involves shoulder depression, shoulder retraction, and shoulder adduction. When a muscle has a high level of stiffness, you should use very few simultaneous opposite movements (for example, to stretch a very tight pectoralis major, you would start by doing shoulder extension and external rotation). As a muscle becomes loose, you can incorporate more simultaneous opposite movements.

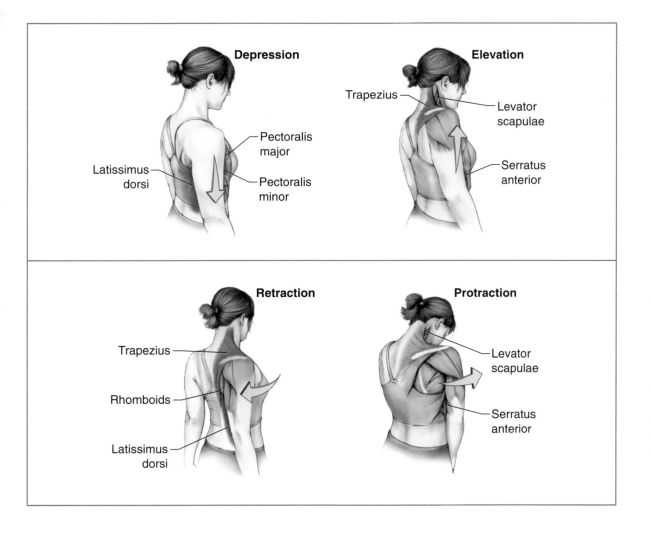

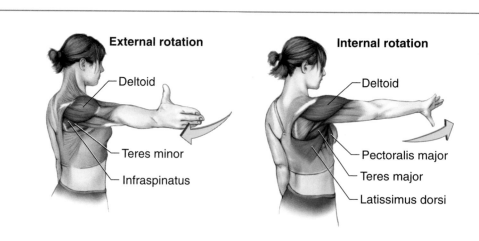

External rotation

— Deltoid

— Teres minor

— Infraspinatus

Internal rotation

— Deltoid

— Pectoralis major

— Teres major

— Latissimus dorsi

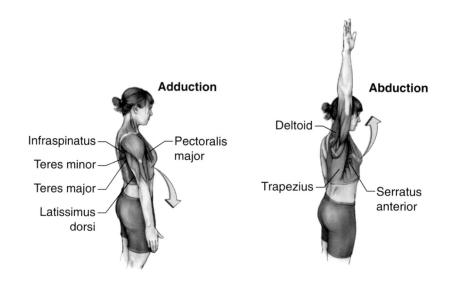

Adduction

Infraspinatus —

Teres minor —

Teres major —

Latissimus — dorsi

Pectoralis major

Abduction

Deltoid —

Trapezius —

— Serratus anterior

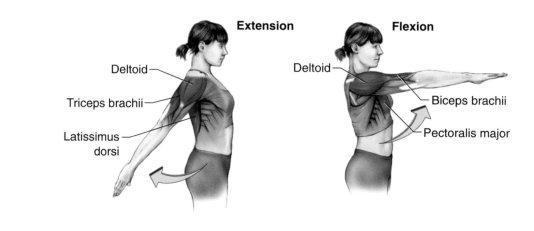

Extension

Deltoid —

Triceps brachii —

Latissimus — dorsi

Flexion

Deltoid —

— Biceps brachii

— Pectoralis major

Muscle	Elevation	Depression	Protraction	Retraction	External rotation	Internal rotation	Abduction	Adduction	Flexion	Extension
Biceps brachii									✔	
Coracobrachialis								✔	✔	
Deltoid					✔	✔	✔		✔	✔
Infraspinatus					✔			✔		
Latissimus dorsi		✔		✔		✔		✔		✔
Levator scapulae	✔		✔							
Pectoralis major		✔				✔		✔	✔	
Pectoralis minor		✔	✔							
Rhomboids				✔						
Serratus anterior	✔		✔				✔			
Subclavius		✔								
Subscapularis						✔				
Supraspinatus							✔			
Teres major						✔		✔		✔
Teres minor					✔			✔		✔
Trapezius	✔			✔			✔			
Triceps brachii										✔

The major joint of the arm, the elbow, is a hinge and thus has only the capacity to either flex or extend. As a result, the muscles that flex the elbow (biceps brachii, brachialis, brachioradialis, pronator teres) are located anteriorly, whereas the extensor muscles (anconeus, triceps brachii) are located posteriorly. The forearm contains two bones: radius and ulna. The radius gets its name from its ability to roll over the ulna, and this ability allows the palm to face either forward (supinated) or backward (pronated). There are two muscles that supinate (biceps brachii and supinator) and two muscles that pronate (pronator teres and pronator quadratus). The pronator muscles are located so that they can pull the radius toward the center of the body, and the supinator muscles are situated to pull the radius away from the body. Interestingly, most of the muscles that control wrist, hand, and finger movements are located at or near the elbow. This results in the belly of the muscle lying near the elbow with tendons crossing the wrist and attaching to the wrist (carpal), hand (metacarpal), and finger bones. Having only tendons in the wrists and hands prevents the wrists and hands from getting too bulky from the increase in size that accompanies muscle strength. Similar to the muscles that move the elbow, all of the wrist flexors (flexor carpi radialis, flexor carpi ulnaris, and palmaris longus) and most of the finger flexors (flexor digitorum profundus, flexor digitorum superficialis, and flexor pollicis longus) are located in the anterior compartment of the forearm. In contrast, all of the wrist extensors (extensor carpi radialis brevis, extensor carpi radialis longus, extensor carpi ulnaris, extensor digitorum communis) and finger extensors (extensor digitorum communis, extensor digiti minimi, extensor indicis) are located in the posterior compartment of the forearm. The muscles that run along the radius (which have *radialis* in their name) do ulnar deviation, whereas those along the ulna (which have *ulnaris* in their name) do radial deviation. Just before crossing the wrist, the tendons of these muscles are anchored firmly by thick tissue bands called the flexor retinacula and extensor retinacula. By passing under the retinacula at the carpal (wrist bones), the tendons lie in a carpal tunnel. Since the tendons are crowded together, each tendon is surrounded by a slippery sheath to minimize friction. Illustrations showing these muscles as well as a chart showing specific movements for each muscle are located at the end of the chapter (pages 50-52).

Stretching the muscles that move the elbows and wrists is helpful in alleviating and sometimes preventing overuse injuries. Because it is more resistive to opposing movements, a tight muscle is easy to damage. When the wrist extensor muscles are tight, pain arises on the medial (close to the body) side of the elbow. In sports, this pain is sometimes referred to as "tennis elbow." Tight wrist flexor muscles, on the other hand, can cause pain on the opposite, or lateral, side of the elbow. This pain is frequently called "golf elbow." Also, constant wrist hyperextension can lead to overstretched tendons in the carpal tunnel. This causes the wrist flexor muscles to tighten, and the constant contraction can lead to increased friction, inflammation, and overuse injury (carpal tunnel syndrome). Continuous stretching of the wrist flexors can strengthen the tendons and help alleviate future problems.

Many of the instructions and illustrations in this chapter are given for either the left or right side of the body. Similar but opposite procedures would be used for the opposite (not pictured) side of the body.

Elbow Flexor Stretch

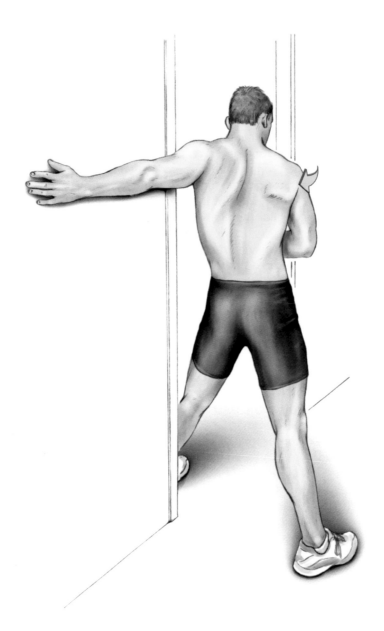

Technique

Stand in a doorway.

While keeping the arm straight, raise the left arm to shoulder level.

Place the arm and palm against the wall with the thumb pointing up.

Rotate the trunk backward toward the wall.

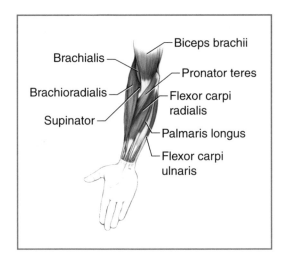

Muscles Stretched

Most-stretched muscles: Left brachialis, left brachioradialis, left biceps brachii.

Lesser-stretched muscles: Left supinator, left pronator teres, left flexor carpi radialis, left flexor carpi ulnaris, left palmaris longus.

Commentary

This stretch is easier to do by grasping a solidly fixed vertical pole. A tight grasp, however, virtually eliminates the stretch effect on the lesser-stretched muscles. Also, it is more difficult to keep the elbow straight, and a straight elbow is necessary for this stretch to be effective. Although it is preferable to lift the arm to shoulder level, the stretch will be effective at whatever height the arm is raised.

Elbow Extensor (Triceps Brachii) Stretch

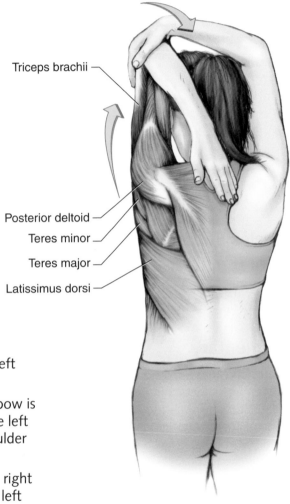

Triceps brachii

Posterior deltoid

Teres minor

Teres major

Latissimus dorsi

Technique

Sit or stand upright with the left arm flexed at the elbow.

Raise the left arm until the elbow is next to the left ear and the left hand is near the right shoulder blade.

Grasp the left elbow with the right hand and pull or push the left elbow behind the head and toward the floor.

Muscles Stretched

Most-stretched muscle: Left triceps brachii.

Lesser-stretched muscles: Left latissimus dorsi, left teres major, left teres minor, left posterior deltoid.

Commentary

Doing this stretch while seated in a chair with a back allows better control of balance. A greater stretching force can be applied to the muscles when the body is balanced.

Elbow Extensor (Anconeus) Stretch

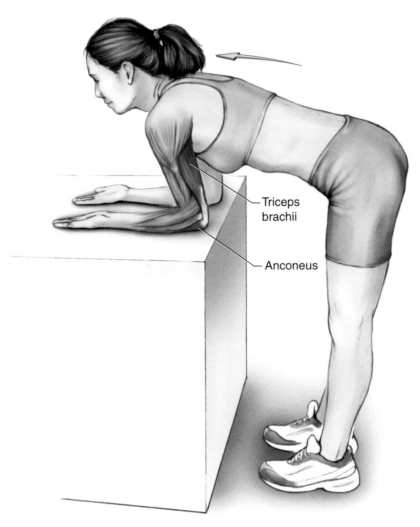

Triceps brachii

Anconeus

Technique

Stand or sit upright while facing a table.

Flex the elbows and rest the forearms on the table with the palms up.

Lean forward, bringing the chest toward the table.

Muscles Stretched

Most-stretched muscle: Left anconeus.

Lesser-stretched muscle: Left triceps brachii.

Commentary

For the greatest stretch, keep the forearms and elbows flat on the table.

Forearm Pronator Stretch

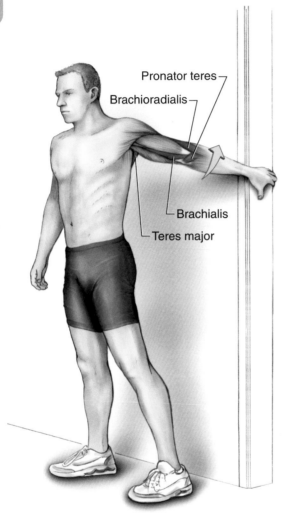

Pronator teres
Brachioradialis
Brachialis
Teres major

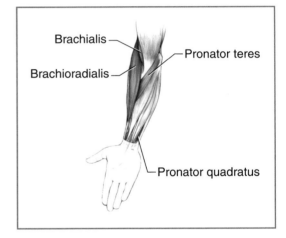

Brachialis
Brachioradialis
Pronator teres
Pronator quadratus

Technique

Stand with the back toward the inside of the doorframe.

While keeping the arm straight, hyperextend the left arm above the midpoint between the hip and shoulder.

Grasp the doorframe with the left hand with the thumb pointing down.

Externally rotate the arm (roll the biceps toward the top).

Muscles Stretched

Most-stretched muscle: Left pronator teres.

Lesser-stretched muscles: Left brachialis, left brachioradialis, left pronator quadratus, left subscapularis, left teres major.

Commentary

You can also do this exercise with a firmly planted vertical pole. To maximize the stretch, keep the elbow straight. After rolling the biceps upward, you can enhance the stretch by inwardly rotating the back toward the hyperextended arm (see figure).

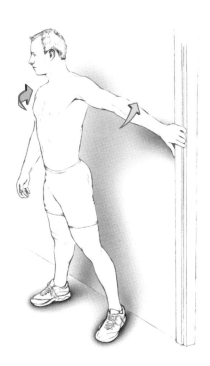

Forearm Supinator Stretch

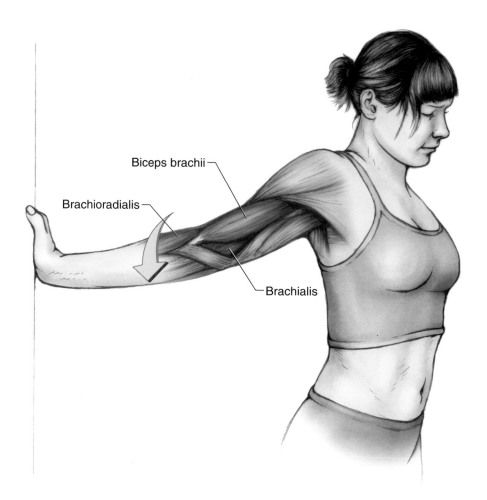

Technique

- Stand with the back toward the inside of the door-frame.
- While keeping the arm straight, hyperextend the right arm above the mid-point between the hip and shoulder.
- Grasp the doorframe with the right hand with the thumb pointing up.
- Internally rotate the arm (roll the biceps down).

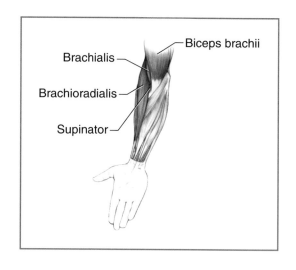

Muscles Stretched

Most-stretched muscles: Right biceps brachii, right supinator.

Lesser-stretched muscles: Right brachialis, right brachioradialis, right infraspinatus, right teres minor.

Commentary

You can also do this exercise with a firmly planted vertical pole. To maximize the stretch, keep the elbow straight. After rolling the biceps downward, you can enhance the stretch by inwardly rotating the back toward the hyperextended arm (see figure).

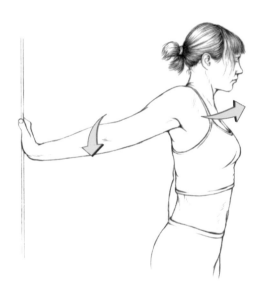

Wrist Extensor Stretch

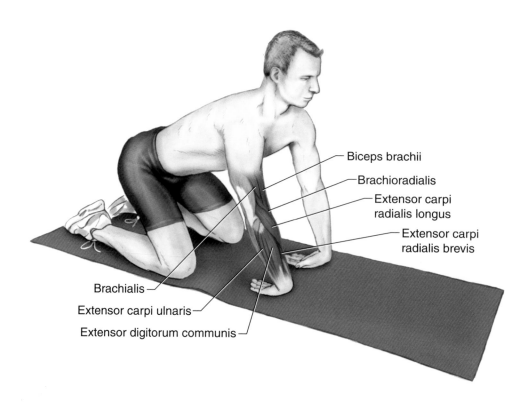

Biceps brachii

Brachioradialis

Extensor carpi radialis longus

Extensor carpi radialis brevis

Brachialis

Extensor carpi ulnaris

Extensor digitorum communis

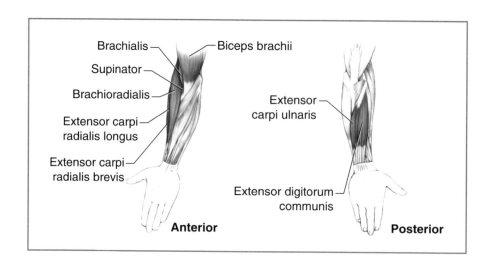

Brachialis

Supinator

Brachioradialis

Extensor carpi radialis longus

Extensor carpi radialis brevis

Biceps brachii

Extensor carpi ulnaris

Extensor digitorum communis

Anterior

Posterior

Technique

Kneel on the floor.

Flex both wrists and place the back of each hand on the floor, shoulder-width apart.

Point the fingers toward the knees.

While keeping the elbows straight, lean backward (buttocks to the heels), keeping the backs of the hands on the floor.

Muscles Stretched

Most-stretched muscles: Brachioradialis, extensor carpi radialis brevis, extensor carpi radialis longus, extensor carpi ulnaris.

Lesser-stretched muscles: Supinator, brachialis, biceps brachii, extensor digitorum communis.

Commentary

The closer the hands are to the knees, the easier it is to keep the backs of the hands touching the floor. The farther the hands are in front of the knees, however, the greater the applied stretch.

Wrist Ulnar Deviator and Extensor Stretch

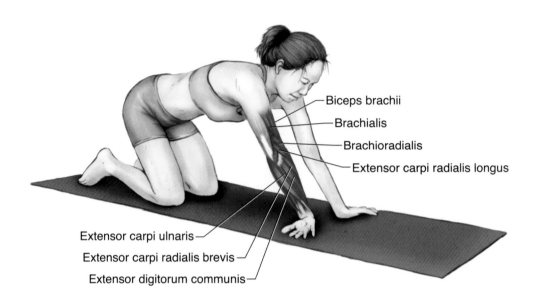

- Biceps brachii
- Brachialis
- Brachioradialis
- Extensor carpi radialis longus
- Extensor carpi ulnaris
- Extensor carpi radialis brevis
- Extensor digitorum communis

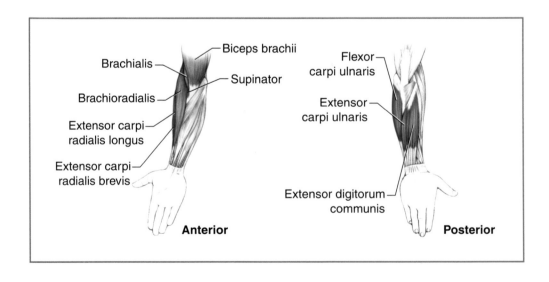

Brachialis
Biceps brachii
Supinator
Brachioradialis
Extensor carpi radialis longus
Extensor carpi radialis brevis

Anterior

Flexor carpi ulnaris
Extensor carpi ulnaris
Extensor digitorum communis

Posterior

Technique

Kneel on the floor.

Flex both wrists and place the back of each hand on the floor.

Point the fingers laterally on a line perpendicular to the midline of the body (the fingertips of the opposing hands pointing away from each other).

While keeping the elbows straight, lean backward (buttocks to the heels), keeping the backs of the hands on the floor.

Muscles Stretched

Most-stretched muscles: Extensor digitorum communis, extensor pollicis brevis, extensor carpi ulnaris.

Lesser-stretched muscles: Extensor carpi radialis brevis, extensor carpi radialis longus, extensor pollicis longus, flexor carpi ulnaris, brachioradialis, supinator, brachialis, biceps brachii.

Commentary

The closer the hands are to the knees, the easier it is to keep the backs of the hands touching the floor. The farther the hands are in front of the knees, however, the greater the applied stretch. The distance each hand is away from the body's midline also influences stretch intensity. The farther away from the midline, the greater the stretch.

Wrist Radial Deviator and Extensor Stretch

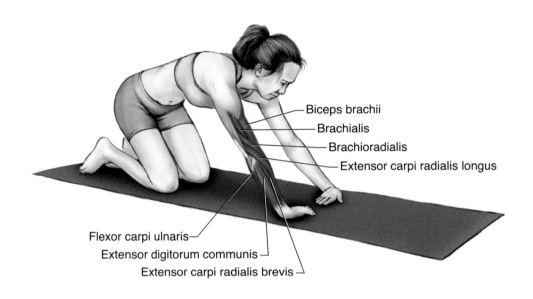

Biceps brachii
Brachialis
Brachioradialis
Extensor carpi radialis longus

Flexor carpi ulnaris
Extensor digitorum communis
Extensor carpi radialis brevis

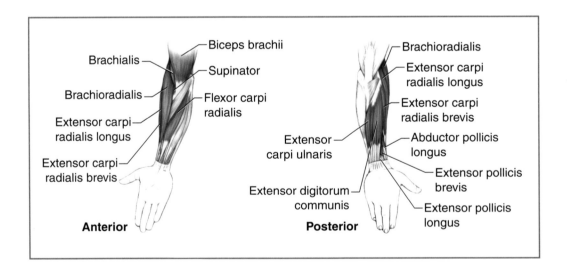

Biceps brachii
Brachialis
Supinator
Brachioradialis
Flexor carpi radialis
Extensor carpi radialis longus
Extensor carpi radialis brevis

Anterior

Brachioradialis
Extensor carpi radialis longus
Extensor carpi radialis brevis
Abductor pollicis longus
Extensor carpi ulnaris
Extensor pollicis brevis
Extensor digitorum communis
Extensor pollicis longus

Posterior

Technique

Kneel on the floor.

Flex both wrists and place the back of each hand on the floor.

Point the fingers medially (the fingertips of the opposing hands pointing toward each other).

While keeping the elbows straight, lean backward (buttocks to the heels), keeping the backs of the hands on the floor.

Muscles Stretched

Most-stretched muscles: Extensor carpi radialis brevis, extensor carpi radialis longus, extensor digitorum communis, extensor pollicis brevis.

Lesser-stretched muscles: Extensor carpi ulnaris, flexor carpi radialis, supinator, brachialis, biceps brachii, brachioradialis.

Commentary

The closer the hands are to the knees, the easier it is to keep the backs of the hands touching the floor. The farther the hands are in front of the knees, however, the greater the applied stretch. The distance each hand is away from the body's midline also influences stretch intensity. The farther away from the midline, the greater the stretch.

Wrist Flexor Stretch

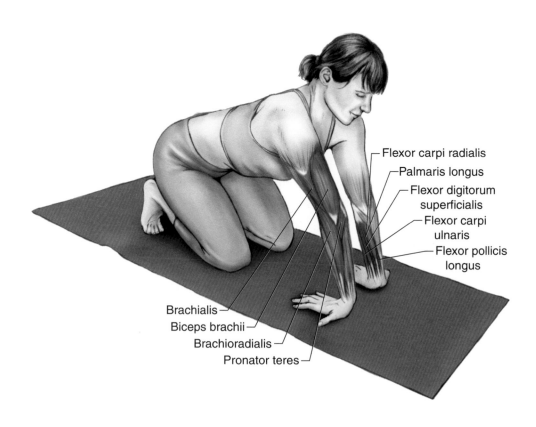

Flexor carpi radialis
Palmaris longus
Flexor digitorum superficialis
Flexor carpi ulnaris
Flexor pollicis longus

Brachialis
Biceps brachii
Brachioradialis
Pronator teres

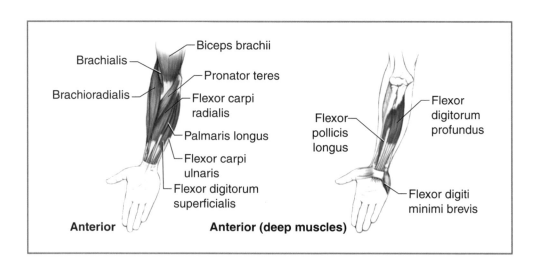

Biceps brachii
Brachialis
Brachioradialis
Pronator teres
Flexor carpi radialis
Palmaris longus
Flexor carpi ulnaris
Flexor digitorum superficialis

Anterior

Flexor pollicis longus
Flexor digitorum profundus
Flexor digiti minimi brevis

Anterior (deep muscles)

Technique

Kneel on the floor.

Flex both wrists and place the palm of each hand on the floor, shoulder-width apart.

Point the fingers toward the knees.

While keeping the elbows straight, lean backward (buttocks to the heels), keeping the palms flat on the floor.

Muscles Stretched

Most-stretched muscles: Brachioradialis, flexor carpi radialis, flexor carpi ulnaris, flexor digitorum profundus, flexor digitorum superficialis, palmaris longus.

Lesser-stretched muscles: Flexor digiti minimi brevis, flexor pollicis longus, pronator teres, brachialis, biceps brachii.

Commentary

The closer the hands are to the knees, the easier it is to keep the backs of the hands touching the floor. The farther the hands are in front of the knees, however, the greater the applied stretch.

Wrist Radial Deviator and Flexor Stretch

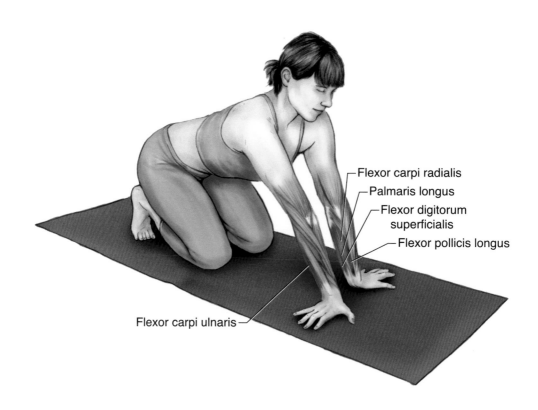

Flexor carpi radialis
Palmaris longus
Flexor digitorum superficialis
Flexor pollicis longus

Flexor carpi ulnaris

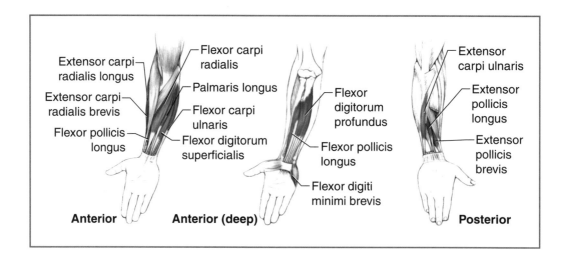

Extensor carpi radialis longus
Flexor carpi radialis
Palmaris longus
Extensor carpi radialis brevis
Flexor carpi ulnaris
Flexor pollicis longus
Flexor digitorum superficialis

Anterior

Flexor digitorum profundus
Flexor pollicis longus
Flexor digiti minimi brevis

Anterior (deep)

Extensor carpi ulnaris
Extensor pollicis longus
Extensor pollicis brevis

Posterior

Technique

Kneel on the floor.

Flex both wrists, and place the palm of each hand on the floor.

Point the fingers outward on a line perpendicular to the midline of the body.

While keeping the elbows straight, lean backward (buttocks to the heels), keeping the palms flat on the floor.

Muscles Stretched

Most-stretched muscles: Flexor carpi radialis, flexor digitorum profundus, flexor digitorum superficialis, palmaris longus.

Lesser-stretched muscles: Flexor carpi ulnaris, flexor digiti minimi brevis, flexor pollicis longus, extensor carpi radialis brevis, extensor carpi radialis longus, extensor pollicis brevis.

Commentary

The closer the hands are to the knees, the easier it is to keep the palms on the floor. The farther the hands are in front of the knees, however, the greater the applied stretch. The distance each hand is away from the body's midline also influences stretch intensity. The farther away from the midline, the greater the stretch.

Wrist Ulnar Deviator and Flexor Stretch

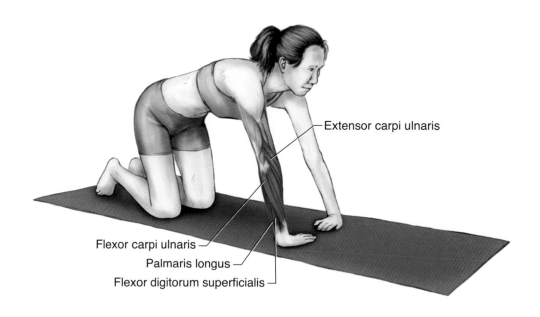

Extensor carpi ulnaris

Flexor carpi ulnaris

Palmaris longus

Flexor digitorum superficialis

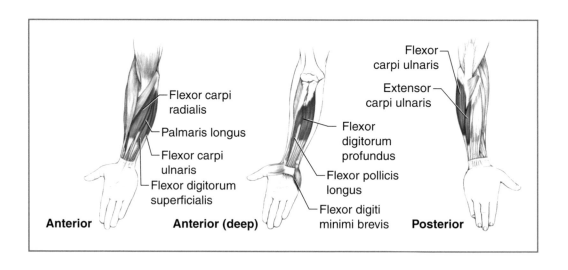

Flexor carpi radialis

Palmaris longus

Flexor carpi ulnaris

Flexor digitorum superficialis

Anterior

Flexor digitorum profundus

Flexor pollicis longus

Flexor digiti minimi brevis

Anterior (deep)

Flexor carpi ulnaris

Extensor carpi ulnaris

Posterior

Technique

Kneel on the floor.

Flex both wrists, and place the palm of each hand on the floor.

Point the fingers medially (the fingertips of the opposing hands pointing toward each other).

While keeping the elbows straight, lean backward (buttocks to the heels), keeping the palms on the floor.

Muscles Stretched

Most-stretched muscles: Flexor carpi ulnaris, flexor digitorum profundus, flexor digitorum superficialis, palmaris longus.

Lesser-stretched muscles: Flexor carpi radialis, flexor digiti minimi brevis, flexor pollicis longus, extensor carpi ulnaris.

Commentary

The closer the hands are to the knees, the easier it is to keep the palms on the floor. The farther the hands are in front of the knees, however, the greater the applied stretch. The distance each hand is away from the body's midline also influences stretch intensity. The farther away from the midline, the greater the stretch.

Finger Flexor Stretch

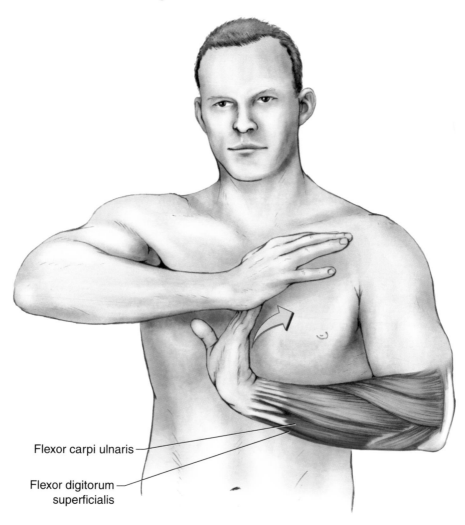

Flexor carpi ulnaris

Flexor digitorum superficialis

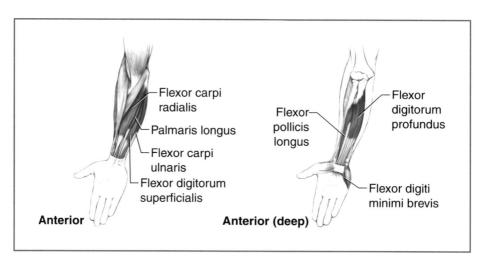

Flexor carpi radialis

Palmaris longus

Flexor carpi ulnaris

Flexor digitorum superficialis

Anterior

Flexor pollicis longus

Flexor digitorum profundus

Flexor digiti minimi brevis

Anterior (deep)

Technique

Sit or stand upright.

Flex the elbow at a 90-degree angle, and extend the wrist as far as possible.

Point the fingers upward.

With the right hand, push the fingers on the left hand toward the elbow.

Muscles Stretched

Most-stretched muscles: Left flexor carpi radialis, left flexor carpi ulnaris, left flexor digiti minimi brevis, left flexor digitorum profundus, left flexor digitorum superficialis, left palmaris longus.

Lesser-stretched muscles: Left flexor pollicis longus.

Commentary

The elbow angle does not need to be precisely 90 degrees. Choose a comfortable angle. Some people find that fully flexing the elbow makes it easier to push on the hand. With the elbow fully flexed, the push is more downward than across.

Finger Extensor Stretch

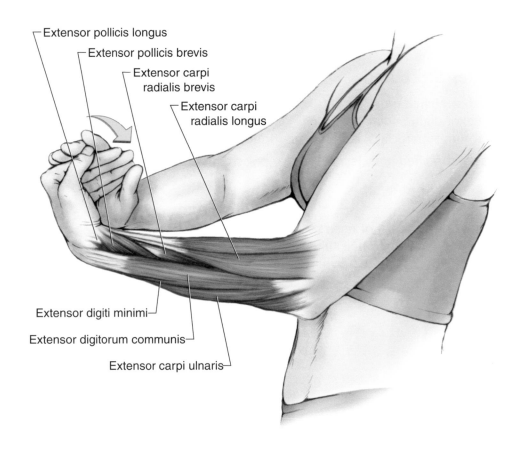

Extensor pollicis longus

Extensor pollicis brevis

Extensor carpi radialis brevis

Extensor carpi radialis longus

Extensor digiti minimi

Extensor digitorum communis

Extensor carpi ulnaris

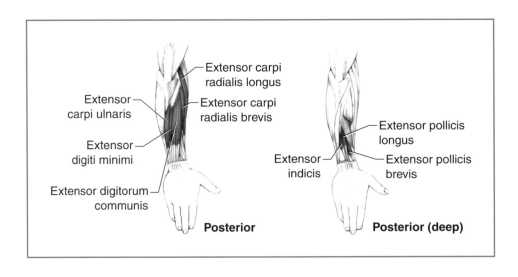

Extensor carpi radialis longus

Extensor carpi radialis brevis

Extensor carpi ulnaris

Extensor digiti minimi

Extensor digitorum communis

Posterior

Extensor pollicis longus

Extensor pollicis brevis

Extensor indicis

Posterior (deep)

Technique

Sit or stand upright.

Turn the left arm so that the palm faces up and flex the elbow to a 90-degree angle.

Flex the wrist to a 90-degree angle, and flex the fingers so that they are pointed toward the elbow.

Place the right hand on top of the fingers and press the fingers down toward the forearm.

Muscles Stretched

Most-stretched muscles: Left extensor carpi radialis brevis, left extensor carpi radialis longus, left extensor carpi ulnaris, left extensor digitorum communis, left extensor digiti minimi, left extensor indicis.

Lesser-stretched muscles: Left extensor pollicis brevis, left extensor pollicis longus.

Commentary

Increase the magnitude of the stretch by flexing the fingers (make a fist). Also, the elbow angle does not need to be precisely 90 degrees. Choose a comfortable angle. Some people find that fully flexing the elbow makes it easier to push on the hand. With the elbow fully flexed, the push is more downward than across.

Arm, Wrist, and Hand Muscle Movements

The stretches in this chapter are excellent overall stretches; however, not all of these stretches may be completely suited to each person's needs. The muscles involved in the various arm and hand movements appear in the table on page 52. To stretch specific muscles, the stretch must involve one or more movements in the opposite direction of the desired muscle's movements. For example, if you want to stretch the flexor carpi radialis, you could perform a movement that involves wrist extension and radial deviation. When a muscle has a high level of stiffness, you should use fewer simultaneous opposite movements (for example, to stretch a very tight flexor carpi radialis, you could start by doing only radial deviation). As a muscle becomes loose, you can incorporate more simultaneous opposite movements.

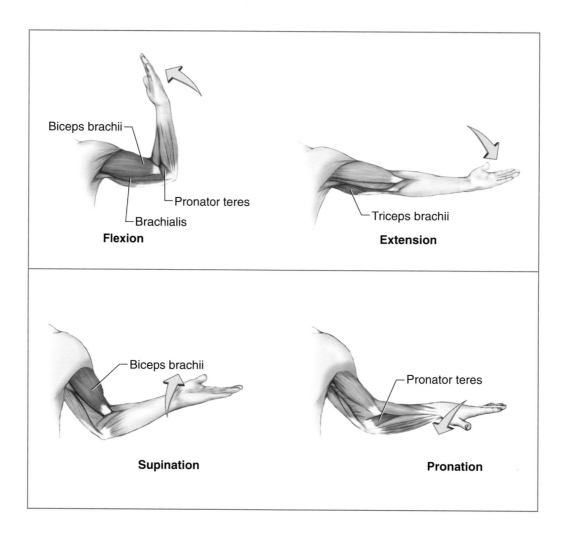

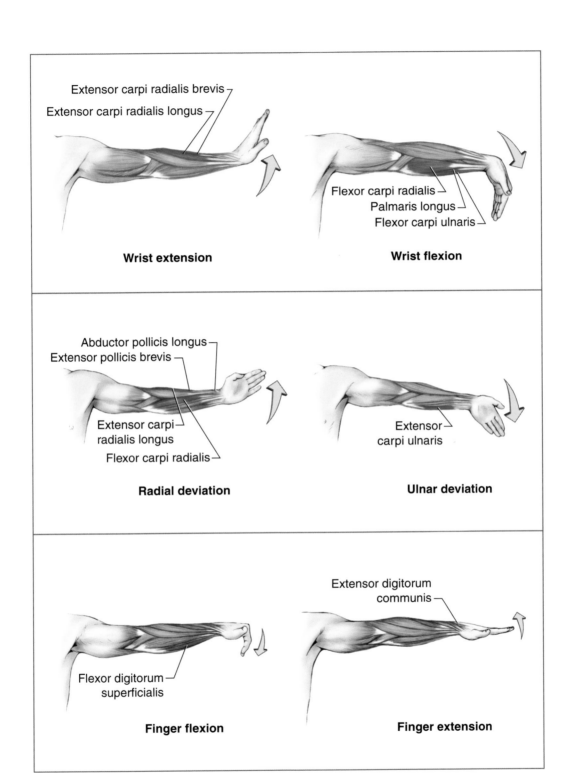

Extensor carpi radialis brevis
Extensor carpi radialis longus

Wrist extension

Flexor carpi radialis
Palmaris longus
Flexor carpi ulnaris

Wrist flexion

Abductor pollicis longus
Extensor pollicis brevis

Extensor carpi
radialis longus
Flexor carpi radialis

Radial deviation

Extensor
carpi ulnaris

Ulnar deviation

Extensor digitorum
communis

Flexor digitorum
superficialis

Finger flexion

Finger extension

ARMS AND WRISTS

Muscle	Elbow flexion	Elbow extension	Pronation	Supination	Wrist flexion	Wrist extension	Radial deviation	Ulnar deviation
Abductor pollicis longus							✔	
Anconeus		✔						
Biceps brachii	✔			✔				
Brachialis	✔							
Brachioradialis	✔							
Extensor carpi radialis brevis						✔	✔	
Extensor carpi radialis longus						✔	✔	
Extensor carpi ulnaris						✔		✔
Extensor digitorum communis						✔		
Extensor pollicis brevis							✔	
Flexor carpi radialis					✔		✔	
Flexor carpi ulnaris					✔			✔
Palmaris longus					✔			
Pronator quadratus			✔					
Pronator teres	✔		✔					
Supinator				✔				
Triceps brachii		✔						

FINGERS

Muscle	Flexion	Extension
Extensor digitorum communis		✔
Extensor digiti minimi		✔
Extensor indicis		✔
Flexor digiti minimi brevis	✔	
Flexor digitorum profundus	✔	
Flexor digitorum superficialis	✔	
Flexor pollicis longus	✔	

Many of the muscles involved in movements of the lower trunk run between the pelvic bones and either the spinal column or rib cage. The abdominal muscles (external oblique, internal oblique, and rectus abdominis) and quadratus lumborum flex the trunk by pulling the rib cage toward the pelvis. On the other hand, the other trunk flexors, iliacus and psoas major, work by either pulling the thigh bone (femur) toward the pelvis (iliacus) or pulling the spinal column toward the femur (psoas major). The prime trunk extensors (iliocostalis lumborum, longissimus thoracis, and spinalis thoracis) are collectively called the erector spinae. The iliocostalis lumborum runs between the posterior pelvis and posterior spinal column, while the longissimus thoracis and spinalis thoracis run along the posterior spinal column and help the individual vertebrae in the spinal column work together as a single unit. The interspinales, intertransversarii, multifidus, and rotatores run between individual vertebrae and cause large movements by making small changes between individual pairs or groups of vertebrae. Figures showing these muscles as well as a chart showing specific movements for each muscle are located at the end of the chapter (pages 66-67).

Many people have stiff back muscles and have discovered that stretching helps to relieve some of the pain accompanying stiff back muscles. The back muscles (or trunk extensors) are not the only lower-trunk muscles to influence back pain. Often people can find relief from back pain by leaning backward (trunk hyperextension); this action actually stretches the abdominal muscles (trunk flexors). This shows that flexible trunk flexors are also important. Moreover, numerous sporting activities (such as golf, tennis, and throwing sports) require twisting of the trunk. Twisting the trunk involves the trunk extensors, flexors, and lateral flexors. Improved range of motion of all lower-trunk muscles can increase the range of motion in trunk rotation and improve the performance in activities that involve these actions.

Hyperextension (arching) and hyperflexion of the lower back are potentially dangerous, especially if you have weak abdominal, thigh, and buttocks muscles. Furthermore, backward roll movements are potentially dangerous to the cervical spine (neck). Injuries from the former and latter stretches may involve excessively squeezing the spinal discs, jamming together the spinal joints, and pinching the spinal nerves emerging from the lumbar vertebrae. Hence, if you perform these stretches, you should do these more gradually than most of the other stretches. Also, to keep pressure off of the neck when doing back rolls, keep the shoulder blades in contact with the floor.

Remember that overstretching (very hard stretching) causes more harm than good. Sometimes the muscles become stiff from overstretching. Overstretching can reduce muscle tone; when tone is reduced, the body compensates by making the loose muscle excessively tight. So, for each progression, start with the position that is the least stiff and progress to the next position only when, after several days of stretching, you notice a consistent lack of stiffness during the exercise. This means that you should stretch both the agonist and antagonist muscles. Also, remember that although there may be greater stiffness in one direction (right versus left), you should stretch both sides so that you maintain proper muscle balance.

Some of the instructions and illustrations in this chapter are given for the left side or right of the body. Similar but opposite procedures would be used for the opposite side of the body.

Lower-Trunk Flexor Stretch
(Back-Lying Position)

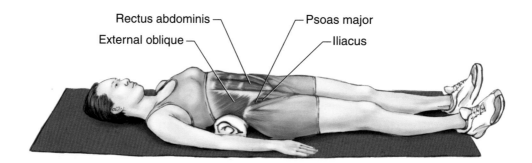

Rectus abdominis — — Psoas major
External oblique — — Iliacus

Technique

Lie on the floor on your back.

Place a rolled-up towel (1 to 2 inches, or 2.5 to 5 centimeters, in diameter) between the small of your back and the floor.

Muscles Stretched

Most-stretched muscles: Rectus abdominis, external oblique, internal oblique.

Lesser-stretched muscles: Quadratus lumborum, psoas major, iliacus.

Commentary

Of all of the stretches in this book that stretch the lower trunk flexors, this stretch is the best for people who have a swayed back or have weak abdominal muscles, since arching the lower back is potentially dangerous for these people. Because the small of the back is supported in this exercise, undesired pressures on the spinal column are reduced. Nevertheless, the width of the back support is important. The larger the diameter of the object, the greater the undesired pressure. Make sure that the upper back, shoulder blades, and buttocks are resting comfortably on the floor. Also, squeezing the buttocks will reduce stress on the lower back.

Lower-Trunk Flexor Stretch
(Front-Lying Position)

Technique

Lie facedown on the floor.

Place both hands palms down; fingers point forward by each hip.

Slowly arch the back, contracting the buttocks.

Continue arching the back and lift your head and chest off the floor.

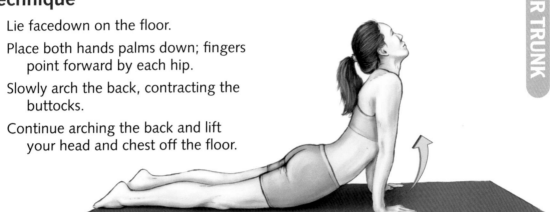

Muscles Stretched

Most-stretched muscles: Rectus abdominis, external oblique, internal oblique.

Lesser-stretched muscles: Quadratus lumborum, psoas major, iliacus, rotatores, intertransversarii.

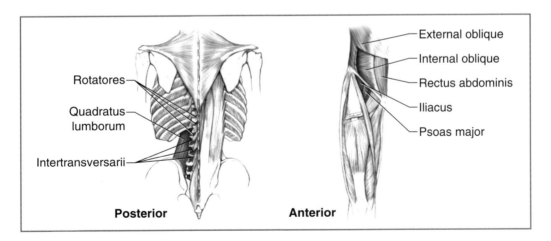

Rotatores

Quadratus lumborum

Intertransversarii

Posterior

External oblique

Internal oblique

Rectus abdominis

Iliacus

Psoas major

Anterior

Commentary

Remember that arching the lower back is potentially dangerous, especially if you have weak abdominal muscles. Injuries from arching the lower back include excessive squeezing of the spinal discs, jammed spinal joints, and pinched spinal nerves emerging from the lumbar vertebrae. Therefore, this stretch is recommended only for those who are very stiff. When doing this stretch, do minimal arching and make sure that you squeeze the buttocks during the arching. Squeezing the buttocks reduces stress on the lower back.

Seated Lower-Trunk Extensor Stretch

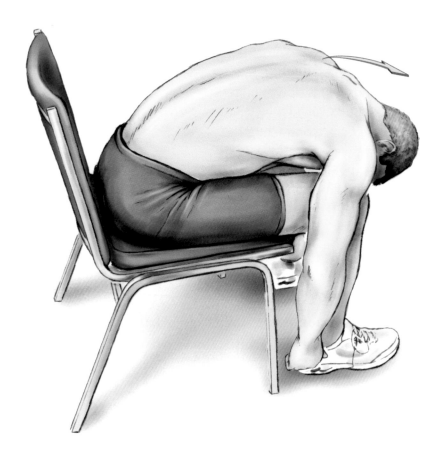

Technique

Sit upright in a chair with legs separated.

Slowly round the upper back and begin to lean forward.

Continue to bend at the waist and lower the head and abdomen between the legs and below the thighs.

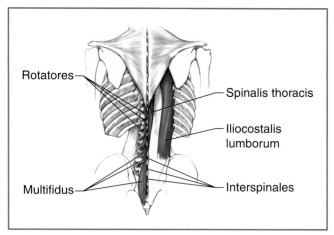

Rotatores

Spinalis thoracis

Iliocostalis lumborum

Multifidus

Interspinales

Muscles Stretched

Most-stretched muscles: Iliocostalis lumborum, multifidus.

Lesser-stretched muscles: Interspinales, rotatores, spinalis thoracis.

Commentary

Remember that hyperflexion can injure the spinal cord. When doing this exercise, go slowly and do not let the back become straight. Also, the effect of the stretch is minimized if the buttocks rise up off of the chair.

Seated Lower-Trunk Extensor Lateral Flexor Stretch

Angling the head toward one of the knees will increase the stretch on the lower-trunk extensors and partially stretch some of the lateral flexors.

Technique

Sit upright in a chair with legs separated.

Slowly extend the upper back and begin to lean forward.

Continue to bend at the waist and lower your head and abdomen toward the right knee.

Slowly lower the head below the right knee.

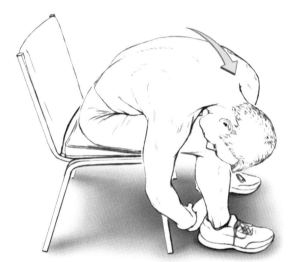

Muscles Stretched

Most-stretched muscles: Left iliocostalis lumborum, left multifidus, left rotatores, left external oblique, left internal oblique.

Lesser-stretched muscles: Left interspinales, left intertransversarii, left quadratus lumborum.

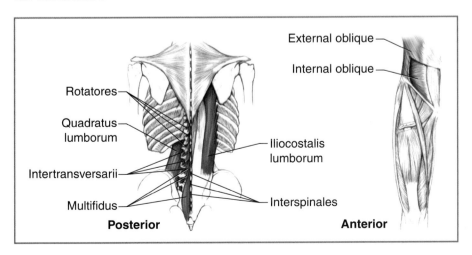

Reclining Lower-Trunk Extensor Stretch

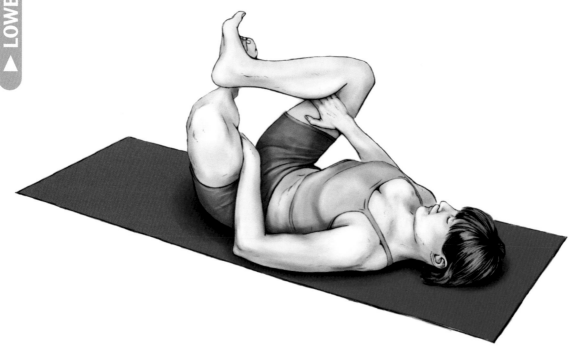

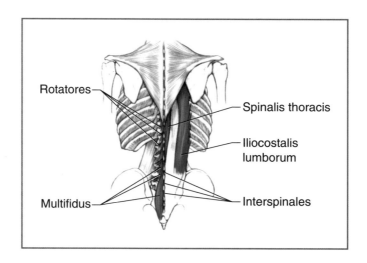

Rotatores

Spinalis thoracis

Iliocostalis lumborum

Multifidus

Interspinales

Technique

Lie on the back with the legs extended.

Flex the knees and hips, bringing the knees up over the chest.

Cross the feet at the ankles and separate the knees so that they are at least shoulder-width apart.

Grasp the thighs at the inside of the knees and pull the legs down to the chest.

Muscles Stretched

Most-stretched muscles: Iliocostalis lumborum, multifidus.

Lesser-stretched muscles: Interspinales, rotatores, spinalis thoracis.

Commentary

Remember that hyperflexion can injure the spinal cord. When doing this exercise, go slowly and do not let the back become straight. To prevent a straight back, allow the spinal column to curl, and raise the buttocks off the floor. Also, do not try to bring the knees too far below the chest (*do not* try to touch the knees to the floor).

Standing Lower-Trunk Lateral Flexor Stretch

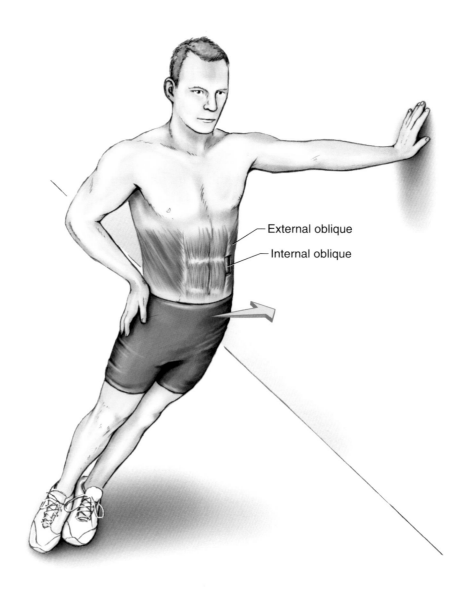

External oblique

Internal oblique

Technique

Stand upright with the feet together and the left side of the body facing a wall about an arm's length away.

Place the palm of the left hand on the wall at shoulder height, and place the heel of the right hand at the hip joint.

While keeping the legs straight, contract the buttocks and slightly rotate the hips in toward the wall.

Use the right hand to push the right hip toward the wall.

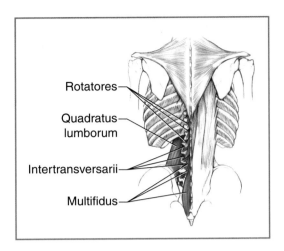

Rotatores

Quadratus
lumborum

Intertransversarii

Multifidus

Muscles Stretched

Most-stretched muscles: Left external oblique, left internal oblique, left rotatores.

Lesser-stretched muscles: Left intertransversarii, left multifidus, left quadratus lumborum.

Commentary

It is very easy to lose balance while doing this exercise, so stand on a nonskid surface. Keep the left arm straight, but do not lock the elbow. You can increase the amount of stretch either by moving the feet farther from the wall, by resting the left forearm on the wall instead of the hand, or both.

Seated Lower-Trunk Lateral Flexor Stretch

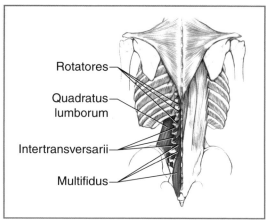

Rotatores

Quadratus lumborum

Intertransversarii

Multifidus

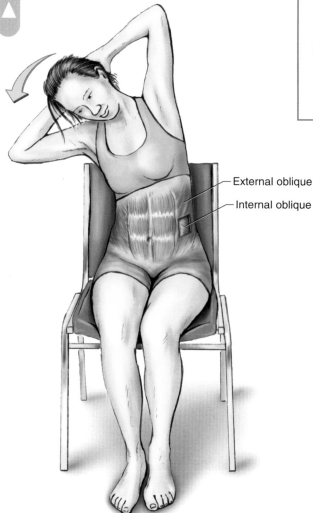

External oblique

Internal oblique

Technique

Sit upright in a chair.

Interlock the hands behind the head, with the elbows in a straight line across the shoulders.

While keeping both elbows back and in a straight line, laterally flex the waist, and move the right elbow toward the right hip.

Muscles Stretched

Most-stretched muscles: Left external oblique, left internal oblique, left rotatores.

Lesser-stretched muscles: Left intertransversarii, left multifidus, left quadratus lumborum.

Commentary

Flexing or extending at the waist will reduce this stretch's effectiveness. Also, keep the buttocks and thighs in complete contact with the chair. The closer the elbow gets to the floor, the harder it will be to remain seated in the chair. Wrapping the lower legs and feet around the chair legs will help in keeping the buttocks and thighs in contact with the seat.

Standing Lower-Trunk Flexor Stretch (Arched Back)

Technique

Stand upright with legs 2 to 3 feet apart (61 to 91 cm) with hands placed on the hips.

Slowly arch the back, contracting the buttocks and pushing the hips forward.

Continue arching the back, drop the head backward, and slide the hands past the buttocks and down the legs.

Muscles Stretched

Most-stretched muscles: Rectus abdominis, external oblique, internal oblique.

Lesser-stretched muscles: Quadratus lumborum, psoas major, iliacus.

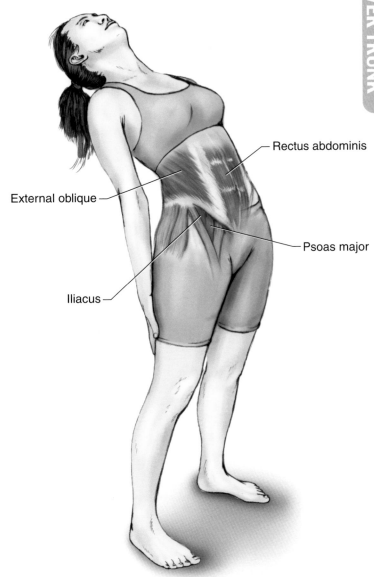

Rectus abdominis

External oblique

Psoas major

Iliacus

Commentary

This exercise is potentially dangerous, especially for those who have a swayed back or weak abdominal muscles. This exercise can worsen a swayed back and cause excessive squeezing of the spinal discs, jammed spinal joints, and pinched spinal nerves emerging from the lumbar vertebrae. This stretch is recommended only for those who are very stiff and do not have a swayed back. Also, you should use this exercise only when the other lower-back flexor stretches do not provide any improvement. When doing this stretch, do minimal arching and make sure that you squeeze the buttocks during the arching. Squeezing the buttocks reduces the stress on the lower back.

Lower-Trunk Lateral Flexor Stretch
(Arched Back)

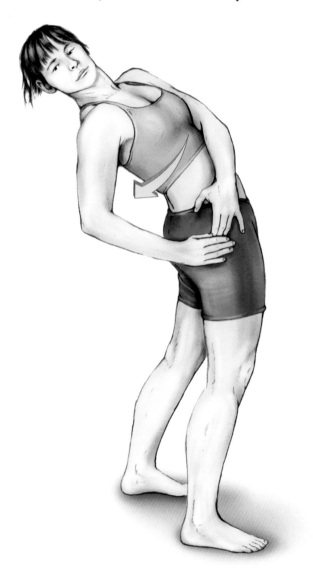

Technique

Stand upright with legs 2 to 3 feet apart (61 to 91 cm) with the right foot about 1 foot (30 cm) ahead of the left foot.

Place both hands near the right hip.

Slowly arch the back, contracting the buttocks and pushing the hips forward.

Continue arching the back, rotate the trunk clockwise, and drop the head back toward the right side.

Slide the hands past the right buttock and down the right leg.

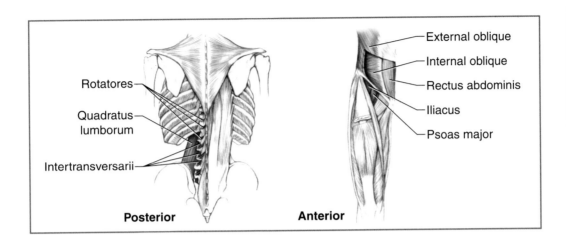

Posterior diagram labels: Rotatores, Quadratus lumborum, Intertransversarii

Anterior diagram labels: External oblique, Internal oblique, Rectus abdominis, Iliacus, Psoas major

Posterior   **Anterior**

Muscles Stretched

Most-stretched muscles: Rectus abdominis, left external oblique, left internal oblique.

Lesser-stretched muscles: Left quadratus lumborum, left psoas major, left iliacus, left rotatores, left intertransversarii.

Commentary

This exercise is potentially dangerous, especially for people with a swayed back or weak abdominal muscles. This exercise can worsen a swayed back and cause excessive squeezing of the spinal discs, jammed spinal joints, and pinched spinal nerves emerging from the lumbar vertebrae. This stretch is recommended only for those who are very stiff and do not have a swayed back. Also, you should use this exercise only when the other lower-back flexor stretches do not provide any improvement. When doing this stretch, do minimal arching and make sure that you squeeze the buttock during the arching. Squeezing the buttock reduces the stress on the lower back. Finally, it is very easy to lose balance while doing this exercise, so take extra care.

Lower-Trunk Muscle Movements

The stretches in this chapter are excellent overall stretches; however, not all of these stretches may be completely suited to each person's needs. The muscles involved in the various lower-trunk movements appear in the following table. To stretch specific muscles, the stretch must involve one or more movements in the opposite direction of the desired muscle's movements. For example, if you want to stretch the left external oblique, you could perform a movement that involves trunk extension and right trunk lateral flexion. When a muscle has a high level of stiffness, you should use fewer simultaneous opposite movements (for example, to stretch a very tight external oblique, you could start by doing only trunk extension). As a muscle becomes loose, you can incorporate more simultaneous opposite movements.

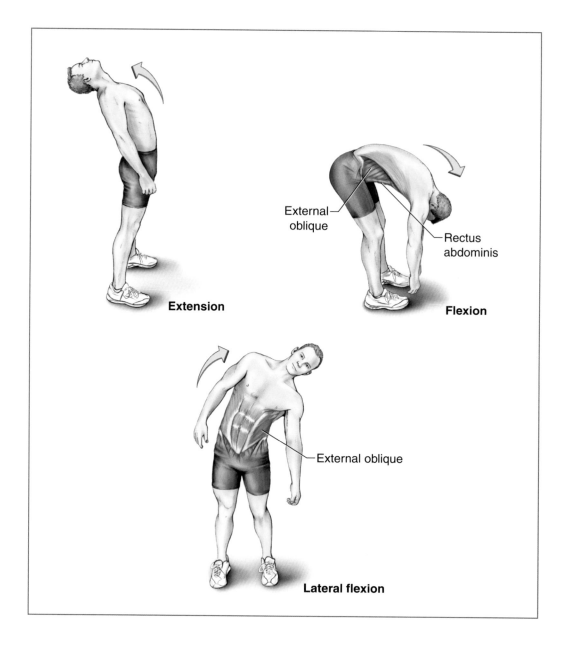

Extension

External oblique

Rectus abdominis

Flexion

External oblique

Lateral flexion

Muscle	Trunk extension	Trunk flexion	Lateral trunk flexion
External oblique		✔	✔
Iliacus		✔	
Iliocostalis lumborum	✔		
Internal oblique		✔	✔
Interspinales	✔		
Intertransversarii			✔
Longissimus thoracis	✔		
Multifidus	✔		✔
Psoas major		✔	
Quadratus lumborum		✔	✔
Rectus abdominis		✔	
Rotatores	✔		✔
Spinalis thoracis	✔		

The hip joint is a ball-and-socket joint, which allows a wider range of muscular movements than most other joints in the body. All but two of these muscles (psoas major and piriformis) run between the pelvic bones and the thigh bone (femur); the psoas major and piriformis run between the lower vertebral column and the femur. The muscles that move the hip joint are some of the most massive muscles (adductor magnus and gluteus maximus) in the body as well as some of the smallest (gemellus superior and inferior). The anterior muscles (psoas major, iliacus, rectus femoris, sartorius) flex the hip and are used during walking to swing the leg forward. The posterior muscles (gluteus maximus, biceps femoris, semimembranosus, semitendinosus) provide the backward swing of walking. A group of large muscles (adductor brevis, adductor magnus, adductor longus, gracilis, pectineus) is on the medial (inside) thigh. These muscles keep the legs centered under the body. A group of small muscles (gluteus medius, gluteus minimus, piriformis, gemellus superior, obturator internus, gemellus inferior, obturator externus, quadratus femoris, tensor fascia latae) is on the lateral (outside) thigh and work to splay the legs to the side. Another group that makes up more than 75 percent of the hip muscles is the external hip rotators (gluteus maximus, gluteus medius, gluteus minimus, piriformis, gemellus superior, obturator internus, gemellus inferior, obturator externus, quadratus femoris, psoas major, iliacus, rectus femoris, sartorius, adductor brevis, adductor magnus, adductor longus, pectineus). Figures showing these muscles as well as a chart showing specific movements for each muscle are located at the end of the chapter (pages 88-90).

Flexibility has more to do with the overall body function than previously thought. For instance, diminished flexibility is one indicator of an aging body. Decreased physical activity also results in decreased flexibility. As people age and decrease their physical activity, they must keep stretching muscle groups in order to maintain mobility and range of motion in the joints. The hip region is located in the middle of the body, so problems in this area tend to radiate and affect many other parts of the body. You can reduce and even prevent many hip problems by paying more attention to strength and joint flexibility.

Often pain in the hip or buttocks area is associated with poor hip flexibility. This is especially true after running or hiking along steep inclines or declines. Hip pain that occurs one to two days after the activity is due to extensive use of the hip external rotator muscles and is caused by damage to both the muscle and the connective tissues in and around the muscle. Stretching these muscles before and after the activity may help decrease this soreness. In addition, the hip external rotator muscles are the least-stretched muscles of the lower body, probably because these muscle groups are also the most difficult to stretch.

Some of the instructions and illustrations in this chapter are given for one side of the body. Similar but opposite procedures would be used for the opposite side of the body.

Seated Hip External Rotator and
Hip Extensor Stretch

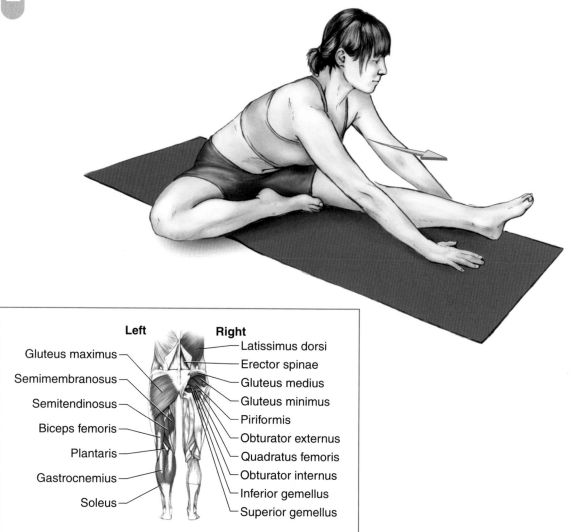

Left	Right
Gluteus maximus	Latissimus dorsi
Semimembranosus	Erector spinae
Semitendinosus	Gluteus medius
Biceps femoris	Gluteus minimus
Plantaris	Piriformis
Gastrocnemius	Obturator externus
Soleus	Quadratus femoris
	Obturator internus
	Inferior gemellus
	Superior gemellus

Technique

Sit on the floor with the left leg extended straight out in front.

Bend the right knee and place the right foot flat against the left inner thigh, as close as possible to the pelvic area.

Place the hands on the floor next to the thighs.

Bend the trunk over toward the left (straight) knee as far as possible until you start feeling a slight stretch (light pain). Keep the left knee down on the floor if possible as you bend over.

As you bend over, reach out with your arms toward the left foot.

Muscles Stretched

Most-stretched muscles on right side: Gluteus medius and minimus, piriformis, gemellus superior and inferior, obturator externus and internus, quadratus femoris, erector spinae, lower latissimus dorsi.

Most-stretched muscles on left side: Semitendinosus, semimembranosus, biceps femoris, gluteus maximus, gastrocnemius.

Lesser-stretched muscles: Soleus, plantaris.

Commentary

Bend the trunk in a forward direction from the hip joint. Keep the trunk as a straight unit; do not let the back curve (see figure below, right). Bending the trunk toward the right knee instead of the left knee reduces the stretch of the most-stretched muscles on the right side of the body and increases the stretch of the most-stretched muscles on the left side of the body.

You can modify this stretch to include the lower-leg muscles (soleus, popliteus, flexor digitorum longus, flexor hallucis longus, posterior tibialis, gastrocnemius, and plantaris). To include these additional muscles, reach out with the left arm, grasp the left foot, and pull the toes slowly toward the knee (dorsiflexed position), as shown in the figure below.

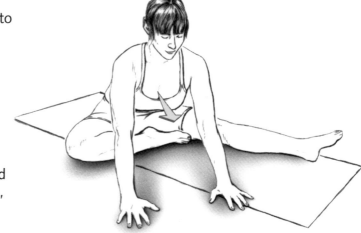

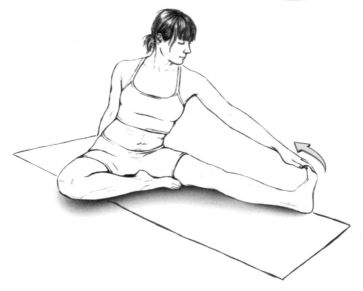

Hip External Rotator Stretch

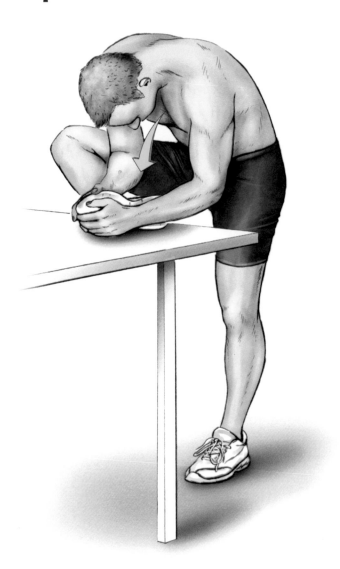

Technique

Stand upright on the left leg with the knee straight; face a support surface (such as a table or beam) that is even with the hips or just a little below the hips.

The right leg is bent at the hip at about a 90-degree angle and rested on the support surface; the outside of the lower right leg rests as flat as possible on the surface. (You can place a towel or pillow under the foot and lower right leg for cushioning.)

Lower the trunk as far as possible toward the right foot, keeping the right knee as flat as possible on the surface.

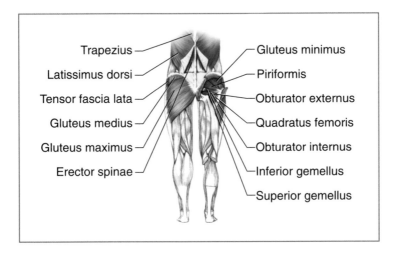

HIPS

Muscles Stretched

Most-stretched muscles: Gluteus maximus and medius and minimus, right piriformis, right gemellus superior and inferior, right obturator externus and internus, right quadratus femoris, lower erector spinae, left latissimus dorsi.

Lesser-stretched muscles: Right tensor fascia lata, right lower latissimus dorsi, lower trapezius.

Commentary

Lower the trunk forward from the hip joint. Keep the trunk as a straight unit; do not let the back curve. Increasing the height of the table, bench, or other surface by 1 to 2 feet (30 to 61 cm) above the hips will increase the stretch on these muscle groups.

Recumbent Hip External Rotator and Hip Extensor Stretch

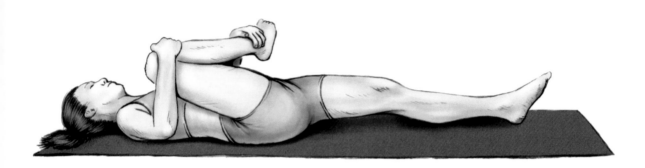

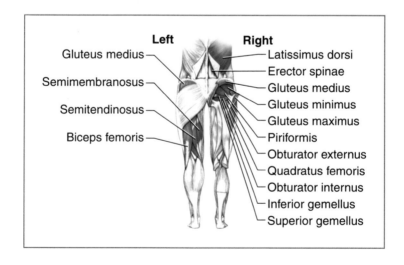

Left	**Right**
Gluteus medius	Latissimus dorsi
Semimembranosus	Erector spinae
Semitendinosus	Gluteus medius
Biceps femoris	Gluteus minimus
	Gluteus maximus
	Piriformis
	Obturator externus
	Quadratus femoris
	Obturator internus
	Inferior gemellus
	Superior gemellus

Technique

Lie on your back on a comfortable surface.

While outwardly rotating the right leg, bend the right knee and bring the right foot to the body's midline (point the knee laterally).

While keeping the left leg flat, grasp the right knee with the right hand and the right ankle with the left hand. Pull the lower leg as a unit as far as possible toward the chest.

Muscles Stretched

Most-stretched muscles on right side of body: Gluteus maximus, gluteus medius, gluteus minimus, piriformis, gemellus superior, gemellus inferior, obturator externus, obturator internus, quadratus femoris, lower latissimus dorsi, erector spinae.

Lesser-stretched muscles in left leg: Semitendinosus, semimembranosus, biceps femoris, gluteus medius (if the leg is kept flat on the floor).

Commentary

Bringing the ankle toward the head or even over the head will stretch the aforementioned muscles to the maximum.

Recumbent Hip External Rotator and Hip Extensor Stretch (Crossed Leg)

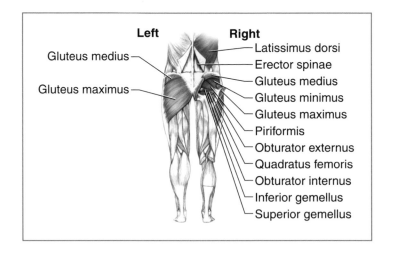

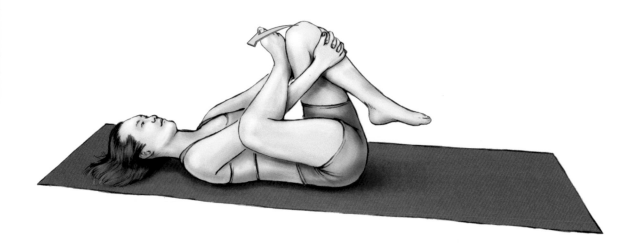

Left   **Right**

Gluteus medius ——
Gluteus maximus ——

— Latissimus dorsi
— Erector spinae
— Gluteus medius
— Gluteus minimus
— Gluteus maximus
— Piriformis
— Obturator externus
— Quadratus femoris
— Obturator internus
— Inferior gemellus
— Superior gemellus

Technique

Lie on your back on a comfortable surface.

Bend the left leg so that the knee is raised up off the floor while keeping the left foot on the floor.

Bend the right knee and cross the right ankle over and just above the left knee.

Grasp the left leg just under the left knee with both hands.

Pull the left knee along with the bent right knee toward your chest as far as possible until you start feeling a slight stretch (light pain).

Muscles Stretched

Most-stretched muscles on right side of body: Gluteus maximus, gluteus medius, gluteus minimus, piriformis, gemellus superior, gemellus inferior, obturator externus, obturator internus, quadratus femoris, lower latissimus dorsi, erector spinae.

Lesser-stretched muscles in left leg: Gluteus maximus, gluteus medius.

Commentary

You can do this stretch while in a sitting position, but it is less effective and more difficult to maintain balance.

Hip External Rotator and Back Extensor Stretch

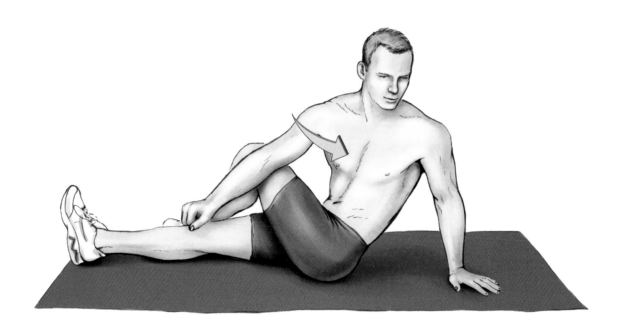

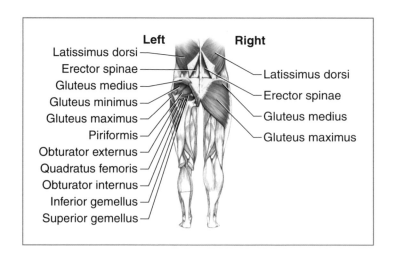

Left		Right
Latissimus dorsi		
Erector spinae		Latissimus dorsi
Gluteus medius		Erector spinae
Gluteus minimus		Gluteus medius
Gluteus maximus		Gluteus maximus
Piriformis		
Obturator externus		
Quadratus femoris		
Obturator internus		
Inferior gemellus		
Superior gemellus		

Technique

Sit on the floor with the right leg extended.

Bend the left leg and place the left foot on the outside of the right knee.

Bend the right arm and position the outside of the right elbow against the outside of the upraised left knee.

Brace the left arm against the floor near the left hip.

Push the right elbow against the left knee, twisting the trunk as far as possible to the left. Maintain enough pressure with the right elbow to keep the left knee in a stable position.

Muscles Stretched

Most-stretched muscles on left side of the body: Gluteus maximus, gluteus medius, gluteus minimus, piriformis, gemellus superior, gemellus inferior, obturator externus, obturator internus, quadratus femoris, lower latissimus dorsi, erector spinae.

Lesser-stretched muscles on right side of body: Gluteus maximus, gluteus medius, erector spinae, lower latissimus dorsi.

Commentary

Do not arch the back or bend forward at the waist.

Hip Extensor and Back Extensor Stretch

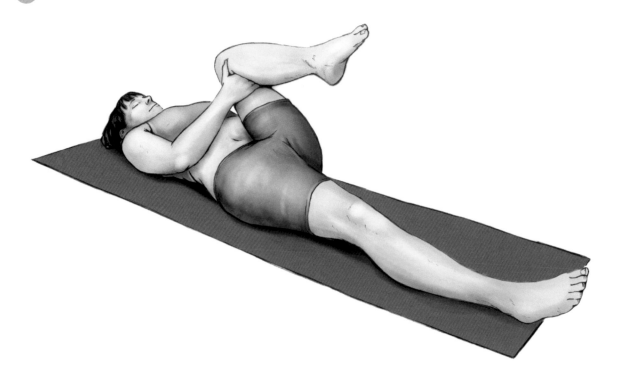

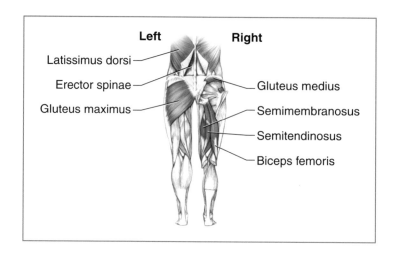

Left	**Right**
Latissimus dorsi	
Erector spinae	Gluteus medius
Gluteus maximus	Semimembranosus
	Semitendinosus
	Biceps femoris

Technique

Lie on your back on a comfortable surface.

Bend the left knee and bring it toward the chest.

While keeping the right leg flat, grasp the left knee with both hands and pull it down toward the chest as far as possible.

Muscles Stretched

Most-stretched muscles: Gluteus maximus, erector spinae, lower latissimus dorsi.

Lesser-stretched muscles in the right leg: Semitendinosus, semimembranosus, biceps femoris, gluteus medius.

Commentary

Bringing the knee toward the armpit instead of the chest will increase the stretch in the muscles. You can do this exercise with both legs simultaneously, but it won't be as effective as when done with each leg separately.

Standing Bent-Knee Hip Adductor Stretch

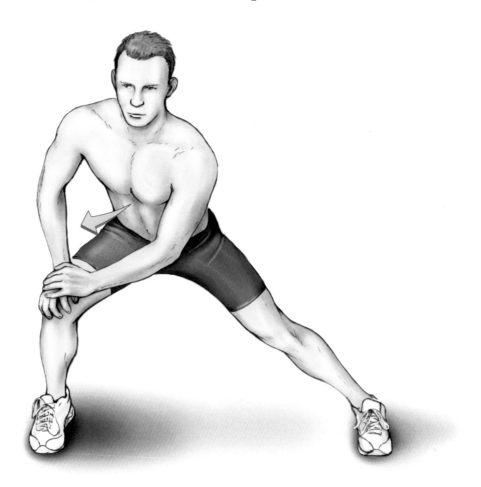

Technique

Stand upright with the legs more than shoulder-width apart and the left foot turned out.

Lower the body (hips) to a half-squatting position, bending the right knee and sliding the left foot outward to the left to keep the left knee straight.

While going down, place the hands on the top of the right knee for support and balance (or hold on to an object for balance).

Muscles Stretched

Most-stretched muscles: Left gracilis, left adductor magnus, left adductor longus, left adductor brevis, left pectineus, middle and lower part of left sartorius, left semitendinosus, left semimembranosus.

Lesser-stretched muscles: Medial side left gastrocnemius and left soleus, left flexor digitorum longus.

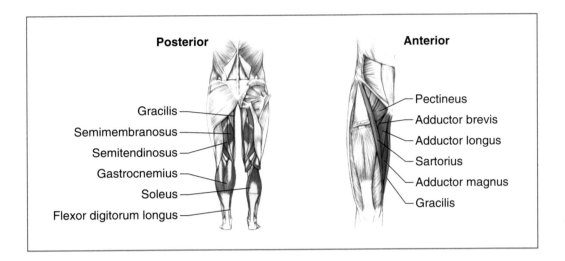

Posterior

Gracilis

Semimembranosus

Semitendinosus

Gastrocnemius

Soleus

Flexor digitorum longus

Anterior

Pectineus

Adductor brevis

Adductor longus

Sartorius

Adductor magnus

Gracilis

Commentary

Keep the trunk as straight as possible. It is more comfortable to rest the left foot on the inside of the foot. To increase the stretch, bend the trunk to the right and press the right thigh down with both hands at the same time.

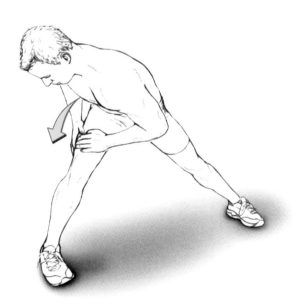

Seated Hip Adductor Stretch

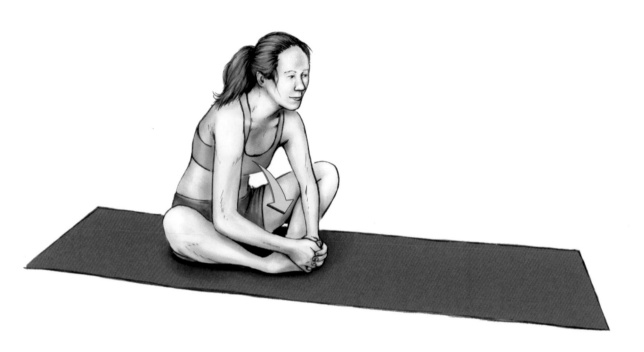

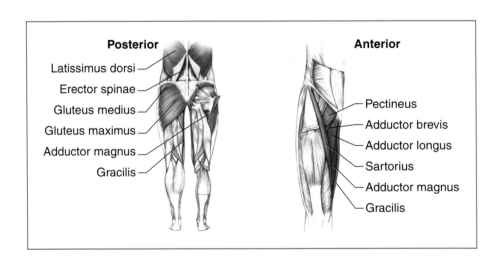

Posterior

- Latissimus dorsi
- Erector spinae
- Gluteus medius
- Gluteus maximus
- Adductor magnus
- Gracilis

Anterior

- Pectineus
- Adductor brevis
- Adductor longus
- Sartorius
- Adductor magnus
- Gracilis

Technique

Sit on the floor in the lotus position (knees bent, feet together with the soles touching).

Bring the heels of the feet as close as possible to the buttocks (distance depends on degree of flexibility).

Grasp the feet or just above the ankles with elbows spreading sideways and touching the legs just below the knees.

Bend the trunk over toward the feet, and press the lower part of the thighs and knees down with the elbows while stretching.

Muscles Stretched

Most-stretched muscles: Gracilis, adductor magnus, adductor longus, adductor brevis, pectineus, middle part of sartorius, lower erector spinae, lower latissimus dorsi.

Lesser-stretched muscles: Gluteus maximus, posterior part of gluteus medius.

Commentary

The closer the heels are to the buttocks, the greater the stretch. Placing the heels 1 foot (30 cm) away from the buttocks increases the stretch on the gluteus maximus, gluteus medius, and erector spinae and places the greatest portion of the stretch on the origins of the adductor muscles.

Standing Raised-Leg Hip Adductor Stretch

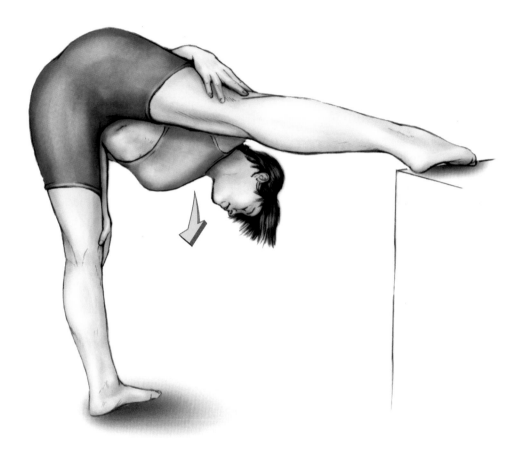

Technique

Stand upright with weight balanced on the left leg.

Place the right leg on a table, bench, or object that is about even with the height of the hips.

While keeping the right knee straight, rotate the body sideways so that the trunk and the left leg face 90 degrees away from the raised right leg (allow the right leg to rotate so that the right knee points to the side). Point the left knee and toes forward (directly in front of the hips).

Bend the left knee slightly, but keep the right knee straight.

Hang both arms down in front of the left leg with the palms close to the floor. Alternatively, place the left hand over the left knee and the right hand on the lateral (outer) side of the right knee (as illustrated).

Bend the trunk slightly forward toward the left knee.

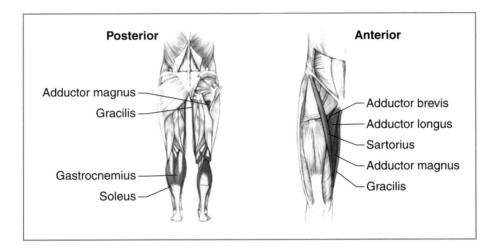

Posterior

Adductor magnus
Gracilis

Gastrocnemius
Soleus

Anterior

Adductor brevis
Adductor longus
Sartorius
Adductor magnus
Gracilis

Muscles Stretched

Most-stretched muscles: Right gracilis, right adductor magnus, right adductor brevis, right adductor longus, right middle sartorius.

Lesser-stretched muscles: Right medial gastrocnemius, right soleus.

Commentary

Make sure to keep the right knee straight. The alternative hand placement allows for greater stretch especially if you apply pressure with the right hand on the right knee. The stretch is also increased with an increased bend of the left knee.

Hip Muscle Movements

The stretches in this chapter are excellent overall stretches; however, not all of these stretches may be completely suited to each person's needs. The muscles involved in the various hip and thigh movements appear in the table on page 90. To stretch specific muscles, the stretch must involve one or more movements in the opposite direction of the desired muscle's movements. For example, if you want to stretch the left adductor magnus, you could perform a movement that involves extension, internal rotation, and abduction of the left leg. When a muscle has a high level of stiffness, you should use fewer simultaneous opposite movements (for example, to stretch a very tight adductor magnus, you could start by doing only hip abduction). As a muscle becomes loose, you can incorporate more simultaneous opposite movements.

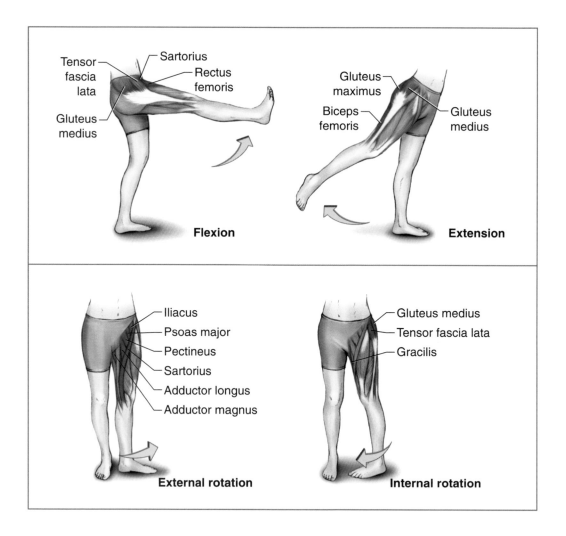

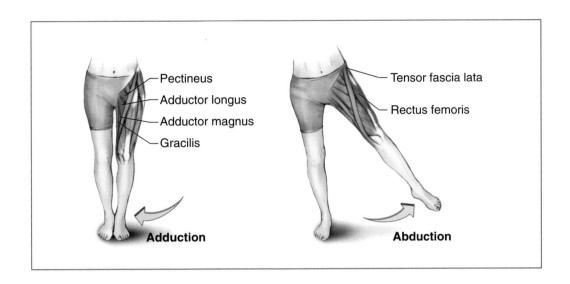

Pectineus
Adductor longus
Adductor magnus
Gracilis

Adduction

Tensor fascia lata
Rectus femoris

Abduction

Muscle	Hip extension	Hip flexion	Hip internal rotation	Hip external rotation	Hip adduction	Hip abduction
Gluteus maximus	✔			✔	✔	✔
Gluteus medius	✔	✔	✔	✔		✔
Gluteus minimus	✔	✔	✔	✔		✔
Biceps femoris	✔			✔		
Semitendinosus	✔		✔			
Semimembranosus	✔		✔			
Rectus femoris		✔				✔
Sartorius		✔		✔		
Pectineus		✔		✔	✔	
Tensor fascia latae		✔	✔			✔
Iliacus		✔		✔		
Psoas major		✔		✔		
Adductor magnus		✔		✔	✔	
Adductor longus		✔		✔	✔	
Adductor brevis		✔		✔	✔	
Gracilis		✔	✔		✔	
Piriformis				✔		✔
Gemellus superior				✔		✔
Obturator internus				✔		
Gemellus inferior				✔		✔
Obturator externus				✔		
Quadratus femoris				✔		

Most of the muscles that control the movements of the knee are found in the thigh. A few calf muscles, however, are also involved. Generally, the thigh muscles that move the knee are categorized into two groups. Four large anterior thigh muscles (rectus femoris, vastus intermedius, vastus lateralis, vastus medialis) are collectively called the quadriceps muscles; these are the major knee extensors. Three large posterior thigh muscles (biceps femoris, semimembranosus, semitendinosus) are collectively called the hamstrings; these are the major knee flexors. The hamstrings are assisted in knee flexion by other thigh muscles (gracilis and sartorius) and a few calf muscles (gastrocnemius, popliteus, plantaris). Figures showing these muscles as well as a chart showing specific movements for each muscle are located at the end of the chapter (pages 110-111).

The muscles of the thigh that control the knee are important in all motor movements. Being much larger than the muscles of the calf and the foot, the thigh muscles are better able to withstand muscular stress. Hence, muscular soreness occurs less often in these muscle groups. It is important, however, to have the right balance of strength and flexibility between the opposing muscle groups of the thigh. Most people have stronger but less flexible quadriceps muscles than hamstring muscles. People tend to stretch the hamstring muscles much more than the quadriceps muscles. This creates an imbalance between the two muscle groups. Chronic overstretching of the hamstrings without comparable stretching of the quadriceps can cause more harm than good. This is the reason hamstring muscles are sore more often than quadriceps muscles. Overstretching can also lead to chronic fatigue and a decrease in strength in the hamstring muscles. To correct this imbalance, you need to put more emphasis on quadriceps stretching and decrease the emphasis on hamstring stretching.

People often sit in one particular position for a long time (as when riding in a car, sitting behind the desk at work, or sitting in an airplane seat). Thus, it is not surprising that people, after sitting for hours, feel the need to get up and stretch their muscles. When people do stand up after long periods of sitting, they typically find that their joints and muscles have become temporarily stiff. Stretching these muscles is a natural remedy. Many have found that stretching provides relief from muscular tension and pain. Since muscular soreness and tension are common in the thigh muscles, both temporary and lasting relief can be obtained from a regular daily stretching routine. This routine needs to be a consistent part of a fitness program.

Most of the instructions and illustrations in this chapter are given for the right side of the body. Similar but opposite procedures would be used for the left side of the body.

Standing Knee Flexor Stretch

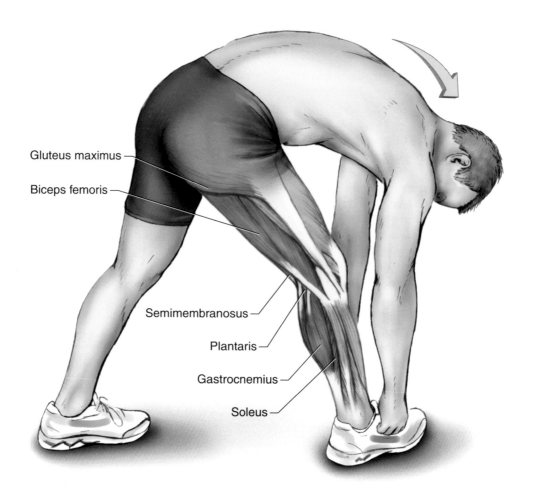

Gluteus maximus

Biceps femoris

Semimembranosus

Plantaris

Gastrocnemius

Soleus

Technique

Stand upright with the right heel 1 to 2 feet (30 to 61 cm) ahead of the left toes.

Keeping the right knee straight and the left knee slightly bent, bend the trunk over toward the right knee.

Reach the hands toward the right foot.

Muscles Stretched

Most-stretched muscles: Right semitendinosus, right semimembranosus, right biceps femoris, right gluteus maximus, right gastrocnemius, lower erector spinae.

Lesser-stretched muscles: Right soleus, right plantaris, right popliteus, right flexor digitorum longus, right flexor hallucis longus, right posterior tibialis.

Commentary

For the best stretch, keep the right knee straight and bend the trunk directly from the hip. Keep the back as straight as possible. Turning the right foot slightly outward and bending the head and trunk more toward the medial (inner) side of the right knee will increase the stretch of the biceps femoris. Turning the right foot slightly inward and bending the head and trunk more toward the lateral (outer) side of the knee will increase the stretch of the semitendinosus and semimembranosus muscles.

Seated Knee Flexor Stretch

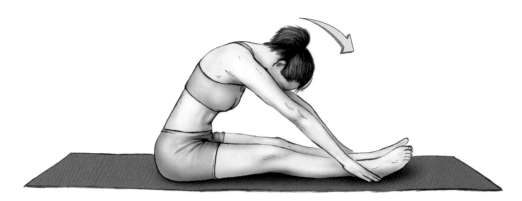

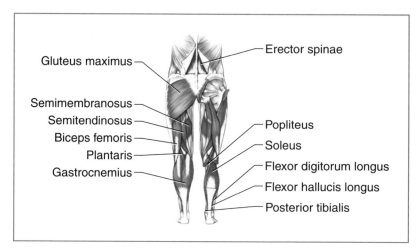

Gluteus maximus
Semimembranosus
Semitendinosus
Biceps femoris
Plantaris
Gastrocnemius

Erector spinae
Popliteus
Soleus
Flexor digitorum longus
Flexor hallucis longus
Posterior tibialis

Technique

Sit on the floor with the legs extended and the inside of the ankles as close together as possible.

Keep the feet relaxed in a natural position.

Place the hands on the floor next to the thighs.

Bend at the waist and lower the head toward the legs. If possible, keep the back of the knees on the floor.

While bending forward, slide the hands toward the feet and keep them alongside the legs.

Muscles Stretched

Most-stretched muscles: Semitendinosus, semimembranosus, biceps femoris, gluteus maximus, gastrocnemius, lower erector spinae.

Lesser-stretched muscles: Soleus, plantaris, popliteus, flexor digitorum longus, flexor hallucis longus, posterior tibialis.

Commentary

To maximize the stretch of the knee flexors, do not bend the knees, tilt the pelvis forward, or curve the back. Also, bend the trunk forward as a single unit, keeping it centered between the two legs.

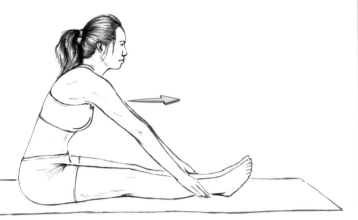

VARIATION

Seated Knee, Ankle, Shoulder, and Back Stretch

Changing the hand position to grasp the toes shifts the stretch to other muscles.

Technique

Sit on the floor with the legs extended and the inside of the ankles as close together as possible.

Keep the feet relaxed in a natural position.

Bend at the waist and lower the head toward the legs. If possible, keep the back of the knees on the floor.

While bending forward, slide the hands toward the feet, grasp the feet, and pull the toes slowly toward the knees (dorsiflexed position).

Muscles Stretched

Most-stretched muscles: Semitendinosus, semimembranosus, biceps femoris, gluteus maximus, gastrocnemius, lower erector spinae, soleus, plantaris, popliteus, flexor digitorum longus, flexor hallucis longus, posterior tibialis.

Lesser-stretched muscles: Lower latissimus dorsi, lower trapezius, posterior deltoid, teres major, teres minor, infraspinatus, triceps brachii.

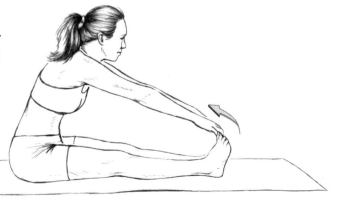

Raised-Leg Knee Flexor Stretch

Technique

Stand upright with weight balanced on the left leg.

Flex the right hip and place the right leg (with the knee straight) on a table, bench, or other stable object that is approximately the same height as the hips.

Bend at the waist, extend your arms over the lower right leg, and lower the head toward the right leg, keeping the right knee as straight as possible.

Keep the left knee straight and the left foot pointing in the same direction as the right leg.

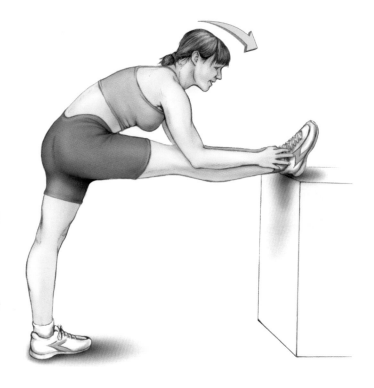

Muscles Stretched

Most-stretched muscles: Right gluteus maximus, right semitendinosus, right semimembranosus, right biceps femoris, erector spinae, lower latissimus dorsi, right gastrocnemius.

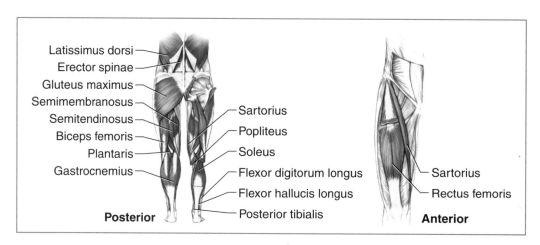

Latissimus dorsi
Erector spinae
Gluteus maximus
Semimembranosus
Semitendinosus
Biceps femoris
Plantaris
Gastrocnemius

Sartorius
Popliteus
Soleus
Flexor digitorum longus
Flexor hallucis longus
Posterior tibialis

Posterior

Sartorius
Rectus femoris

Anterior

Lesser-stretched muscles: Right soleus, right popliteus, right plantaris, right flexor digitorum longus, right flexor hallucis longus, right posterior tibialis, left sartorius, left rectus femoris.

Commentary

To maximize the stretch of the knee flexors, do not bend the knees, tilt the pelvis forward, or curve the back. Also, bend the trunk straight forward as a single unit, keeping it centered over the right leg.

Increasing the height of the table or bench by 1 to 2 feet (30 to 61 cm) above the hips will increase the stretch of these muscle groups. You will also start feeling a stretch in some of the left-side muscle groups (sartorius, rectus femoris, vastus intermedius, lateralis, and medialis) as you increase the height of the table.

VARIATION

Raised-Leg Knee, Ankle, Shoulder, and Back Stretch

Changing the hand position to grasp the toes shifts the stretch to other muscles.

Technique

Stand upright with weight balanced on the left leg.

Flex the right hip and place the right leg (with the knee straight) on a table, bench, or other stable object that is approximately the same height as the hips.

Bend at the waist, extend your arms over the lower right leg, and lower the head toward the right leg, keeping the right knee as straight as possible.

While bending forward, slide the hands toward the feet, grasp the feet, and pull the toes slowly toward the knees (dorsiflexed position).

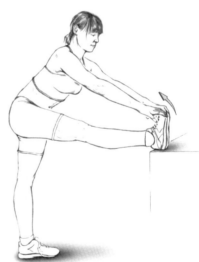

Muscles Stretched

Most-stretched muscles: Right gluteus maximus, right semitendinosus, right semimembranosus, right biceps femoris, erector spinae, lower latissimus dorsi, right gastrocnemius, right soleus, right popliteus, right plantaris, right flexor digitorum longus, right flexor hallucis longus, right posterior tibialis.

Lesser-stretched muscles: Left sartorius, left rectus femoris, lower trapezius, posterior deltoid, teres major, teres minor, infraspinatus, triceps brachii.

Recumbent Knee Flexor Stretch

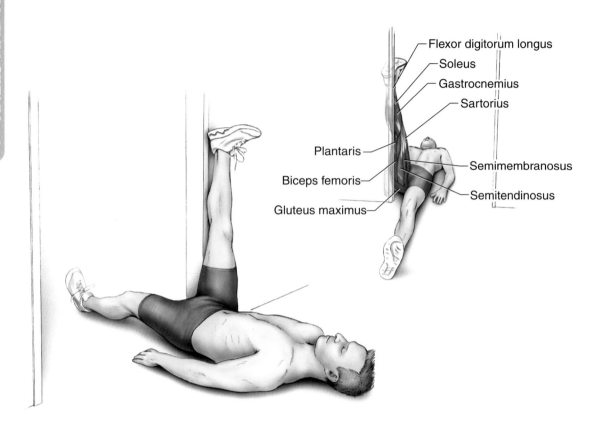

Flexor digitorum longus
Soleus
Gastrocnemius
Sartorius
Plantaris
Biceps femoris
Gluteus maximus
Semimembranosus
Semitendinosus

Technique

Lie flat on your back in a doorway with the hips placed in front of the doorframe.

Raise the right leg and rest it on the doorframe. Keep the right knee straight and the left leg flat on the floor.

Place the hands palms down on either side of the buttocks.

Keeping the right leg straight, use the hands to slowly move the buttocks through the doorframe until you feel a stretch in the back of the leg.

Muscles Stretched

Most-stretched muscles: Right gluteus maximus, right semitendinosus, right semimembranosus, right biceps femoris, right gastrocnemius.

Lesser-stretched muscles: Right soleus, right popliteus, right plantaris, right flexor digitorum longus, right flexor hallucis longus, right posterior tibialis, left sartorius, left rectus femoris.

Commentary

To maximize the stretch of the knee flexors, do not bend the knees, tilt the pelvis forward, or curve the back. Adjust the distance between the buttocks and the doorframe to increase or decrease the stretch. The closer the buttocks are to the doorframe, the greater the stretch. Once the buttocks cannot be positioned any closer to the doorframe, bending the leg at the hip and moving the leg toward the head can increase the stretch.

VARIATION

Recumbent Knee, Ankle, Shoulder, and Back Stretch

Using a towel to bend the toes shifts the stretch to other muscles.

Technique

Lie flat on your back in a doorway with the hips placed in front of the doorframe.

Raise the right leg and rest it on the doorframe. Keep the right knee straight and the left leg flat on the floor.

Place a towel, cloth, or band over and around the toes and grasp both ends firmly with the hands.

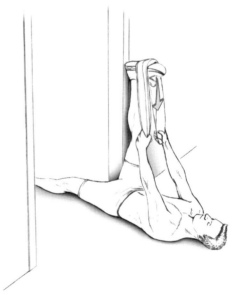

Keeping the right leg straight, place the hands on the doorframe and slowly move the buttocks through the doorframe until you feel a stretch in the back of the leg.

Once you feel the stretch in the back of the leg, use the towel to pull the toes and foot down toward the head.

Muscles Stretched

Most-stretched muscles: Right gluteus maximus, right semitendinosus, right semimembranosus, right biceps femoris, erector spinae, lower latissimus dorsi, right gastrocnemius, right soleus, right popliteus, right plantaris, right flexor digitorum longus, right flexor hallucis longus, right posterior tibialis.

Lesser-stretched muscles: Left sartorius, left rectus femoris, lower trapezius, posterior deltoid, teres major, teres minor, infraspinatus, triceps brachii.

Seated Knee Flexor and Hip Adductor Stretch

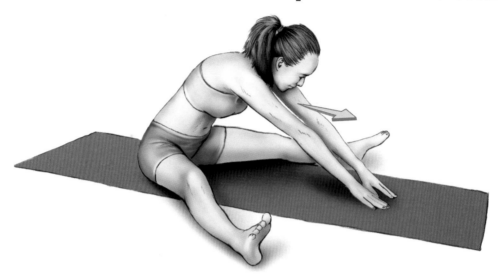

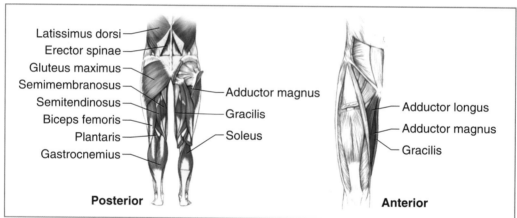

Latissimus dorsi

Erector spinae

Gluteus maximus

Semimembranosus

Semitendinosus

Biceps femoris

Plantaris

Gastrocnemius

Adductor magnus

Gracilis

Soleus

Posterior

Adductor longus

Adductor magnus

Gracilis

Anterior

Technique

Sit comfortably on the floor with legs extended in a V position (feet far apart from each other).

Place the hands on the floor next to the thighs.

Keep both knees straight and as flat against the floor as possible. Reach the hands out toward the center or slide the hands forward along the legs and bend the trunk over between the knees.

Muscles Stretched

Most-stretched muscles: Semitendinosus, semimembranosus, gracilis, adductor magnus and longus, gluteus maximus, lower erector spinae, lower latissimus dorsi, medial side of soleus, medial head of gastrocnemius.

Lesser-stretched muscles: Lateral soleus, lateral head of gastrocnemius, plantaris, biceps femoris.

Commentary

To maximize the stretch, do not bend the knees, tilt the pelvis forward, or curve the back. Also, bend the trunk forward as a single unit, keeping it centered between the two legs.

VARIATION

Seated Knee, Hip, Ankle, Shoulder, and Back Stretch

Changing the hand position to grasp the toes shifts the stretch to other muscles.

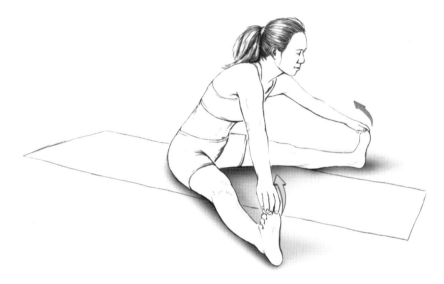

Technique

Sit comfortably on the floor with legs extended in a V position (feet far apart from each other).

Keep both knees straight and as flat against the floor as possible. Slide the hands forward along the legs and bend the trunk over between the knees. At the same time, grasp the toes of both feet and pull them toward the body.

Muscles Stretched

Most-stretched muscles: Semitendinosus, semimembranosus, gracilis, adductor magnus, adductor longus, gluteus maximus, lower erector spinae, lower latissimus dorsi, soleus, gastrocnemius, popliteus, plantaris, flexor digitorum longus, flexor hallucis longus, posterior tibialis.

Lesser-stretched muscles: Biceps femoris, posterior deltoid, triceps brachii, teres major, teres minor, infraspinatus, lower trapezius.

Standing Knee Flexor and Hip Adductor Stretch

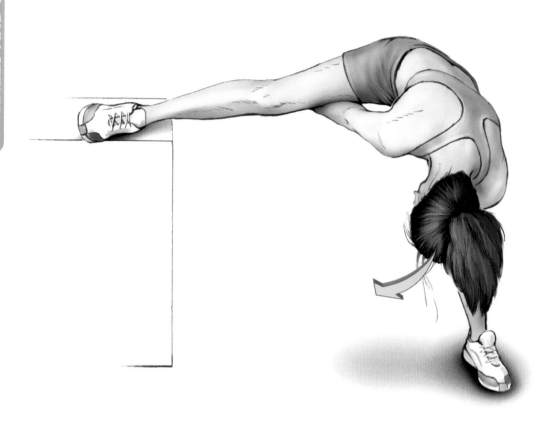

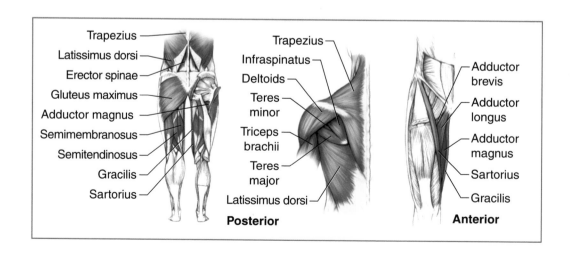

Posterior

Anterior

Technique

Stand with the right side of the body near a table, bench, or object at the approximate height of the hips.

While balancing the weight on the left leg, raise the right leg and position it on the table, bench, or object.

Keeping the knees straight, bend the trunk over between the knees as far as possible.

As you bend the trunk, reach between the knees and place the hands behind the thighs.

Muscles Stretched

Most-stretched muscles: Gluteus maximus, semitendinosus, semimembranosus, gracilis, adductor magnus, adductor brevis, adductor longus, sartorius, erector spinae, latissimus dorsi.

Lesser-stretched muscles: Posterior deltoids, triceps brachii, lower trapezius, teres minor, teres major, infraspinatus.

Commentary

Keep the knees straight, bend the trunk forward from the hip joint, and keep the trunk as a straight unit (no back curve). By increasing the height of the table, bench, or other object 1 to 2 feet (30 to 61 cm) above the hips, you will have additional benefits to the noted muscle groups.

One-Leg Kneeling Knee Extensor Stretch

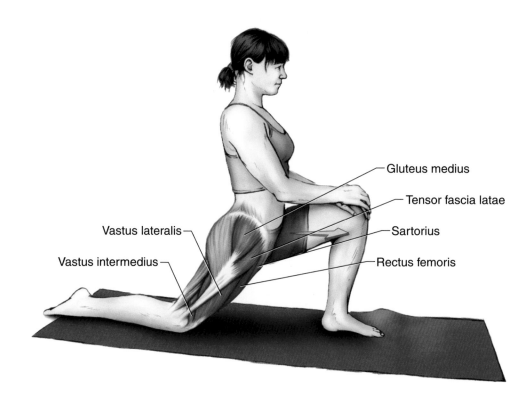

Gluteus medius

Tensor fascia latae

Sartorius

Rectus femoris

Vastus lateralis

Vastus intermedius

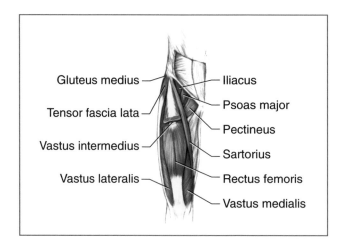

Gluteus medius

Iliacus

Tensor fascia lata

Psoas major

Pectineus

Vastus intermedius

Sartorius

Vastus lateralis

Rectus femoris

Vastus medialis

Technique

Step forward with the left leg and bend the knee at about a 90-degree angle. Keep the left knee positioned above the left ankle.

Extend the right leg behind the torso and touch the floor with the right knee; the lower leg lies on the floor.

Hold on to an object or place the hands on the left knee to maintain balance.

Move the hips forward, pushing the left knee in front of the left ankle and dorsiflexing that ankle.

Muscles Stretched

Most-stretched muscles: Right vastus medialis, right vastus intermedius, right vastus lateralis, middle and upper right sartorius, right rectus femoris, right psoas major, right iliacus, right tensor fascia lata.

Lesser-stretched muscles: Right pectineus, anterior part of right gluteus medius.

Commentary

Move slowly to the stretched position and keep the left knee pointing forward. Do not let the left knee point to either side or let the right knee move along the floor. While the hips are placed in the forward direction, arching the back can increase the stretch on the muscles.

One-Leg Standing Hip Flexor and Knee Extensor Stretch

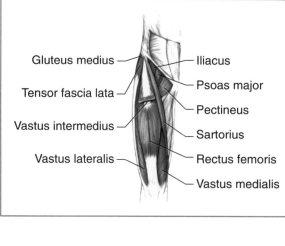

Gluteus medius

Tensor fascia lata

Vastus intermedius

Vastus lateralis

Iliacus

Psoas major

Pectineus

Sartorius

Rectus femoris

Vastus medialis

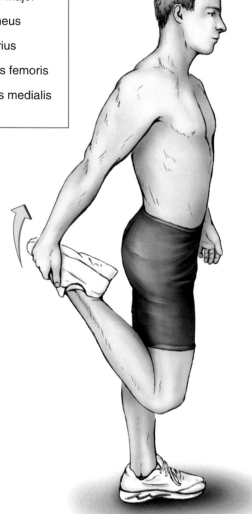

Technique

Stand upright with weight balanced on the left leg. Keep the left foot pointing straight forward and the knee almost straight. To help maintain balance, brace the left hand on a wall.

Bend the right knee; grasp the right foot or ankle tightly and pull the right heel backward and slightly upward to within 4 to 6 inches (10 to 15 cm) of the buttocks.

At the same time, push the hips forward.

Muscles Stretched

Most-stretched muscles: Right vastus medialis, right vastus intermedius, right vastus lateralis, middle and upper right sartorius, right rectus femoris, right psoas major, right iliacus, right tensor fascia lata.

Lesser-stretched muscles: Right pectineus, anterior part of right gluteus medius.

Commentary

When doing this stretch, be extra careful not to strain the knee structure by over-flexing the knee. Pull the ankle slowly in a more backward than upward direction, making sure that the hips also move forward. In other words, concentrate more on doing hip extension than on doing knee flexion. To place most of the stretch emphasis on the medial muscles (vastus medialis and pectineus), rotate the upper body away from the medial muscles (rotate the right side clockwise) when bending backward. To place most of the stretch emphasis on the lateral muscles (vastus lateralis and tensor fascia latae), rotate the upper body away from the lateral muscles (rotate the right side counterclockwise) when bending backward.

VARIATION

Supported One-Leg Standing Hip Flexor and Knee Extensor Stretch

You can also do this stretch by bracing the right foot on a table or beam. Because of the increased possibility of hyperflexing the knee, this is a more advanced stretch; you should do this stretch only if you have very flexible muscles.

Technique

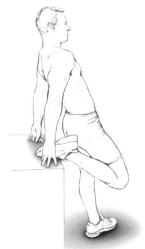

Stand with the back toward a padded table, bed, or soft platform that is below the height of the hips.

Balance the weight on the left leg and bend the knee slightly.

Bend the right knee and prop the right ankle on the rear support surface.

Place both hands on the rear support surface 6 to 12 inches (15 to 30 cm) behind the buttocks.

Move the torso backward slowly so that the heel of the right foot touches the buttocks. Make sure that the ankle and knee are comfortable.

Push the hips forward and simultaneously arch the back by bending the shoulders toward the buttocks.

Muscles Stretched

Most-stretched muscles: Right vastus medialis, right vastus intermedius, right vastus lateralis, middle and upper right sartorius, right rectus femoris, right psoas major, right iliacus, right tensor fascia lata.

Lesser-stretched muscles: Right pectineus, anterior part of right gluteus medius.

Lying Hip Flexor and Knee Extensor Stretch

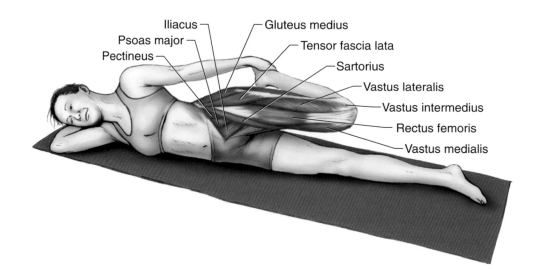

Iliacus
Psoas major
Pectineus
Gluteus medius
Tensor fascia lata
Sartorius
Vastus lateralis
Vastus intermedius
Rectus femoris
Vastus medialis

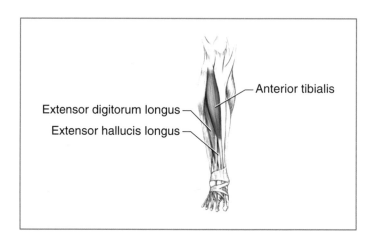

Anterior tibialis
Extensor digitorum longus
Extensor hallucis longus

Technique

Lie on the right side of the body.

Bend the left knee and bring the left heel to within 4 to 6 inches (10 to 15 cm) of the buttocks.

Grasp the left ankle tightly and pull the leg backward close to your buttocks. However, do not bring the heel of the left ankle all the way to the buttocks.

Push the hip forward at the same time.

Muscles Stretched

Most-stretched muscles: Left vastus intermedius, left rectus femoris, left psoas major, middle and upper left sartorius.

Lesser-stretched muscles: Left vastus medialis, left vastus lateralis, left tensor fascia lata, left pectineus, left iliacus, anterior part of left gluteus medius, left anterior tibialis, left extensor digitorum longus, left extensor hallucis longus.

Commentary

When doing this stretch, be extra careful not to strain the knee structure by over-flexing the knee. Pull the ankle slowly in a more backward direction than upward direction, making sure that the hips are also moved forward. In other words, concentrate more on doing hip extension than on doing knee flexion.

Knee and Thigh Muscle Movements

The stretches in this chapter are excellent overall stretches; however, not all of these stretches may be completely suited to each person's needs. The muscles involved in the various thigh and knee movements appear in the following table. To stretch specific muscles, the stretch must involve one or more movements in the opposite direction of the desired muscle's movements. For example, if you want to stretch the left biceps femoris, you would perform a movement that involves extension and internal rotation of the left leg. When a muscle has a high level of stiffness, you should use fewer simultaneous opposite movements (for example, to stretch a very tight biceps femoris, you could start by doing only knee extension). As a muscle becomes loose, you can incorporate more simultaneous opposite movements.

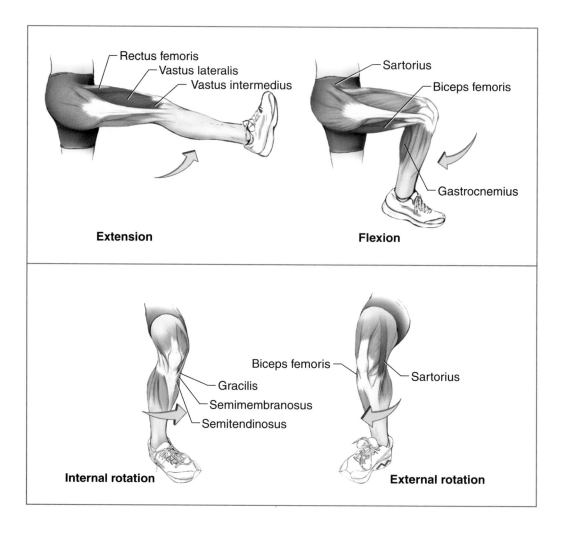

Muscle	Knee extension	Knee flexion	Internal rotation	External rotation
Rectus femoris	✔			
Vastus medialis	✔			
Vastus lateralis	✔			
Vastus intermedius	✔			
Sartorius		✔		✔
Biceps femoris		✔		✔
Semitendinosus		✔	✔	
Semimembranosus		✔	✔	
Gracilis		✔	✔	
Popliteus		✔	✔	
Gastrocnemius		✔		
Plantaris		✔		

The muscles that move the ankle and toes are located primarily in the lower leg and can be described as muscles with tendons as long as or longer than the muscle. The predominant tendon is the Achilles tendon. Three muscles (gastrocnemius, plantaris, soleus) share this tendon, and the three collectively are called the triceps surae. The triceps surae muscles are the prime plantar flexors and are assisted by the popliteus and posterior tibialis as well as flexor digitorum longus and flexor hallucis longus, which also move the toes. Another group of three muscles (peroneus longus, peroneus brevis, peroneus tertius) is located on the outer (lateral) side of the calf; these muscles are used in pulling the inner ankles toward the floor. The anterior calf muscles (anterior tibialis, extensor hallucis longus, extensor digitorum longus) not only dorsiflex the ankle but also move the foot and toes. The muscles on the dorsal (top) side of the foot (extensor digitorum brevis, dorsal interosseous, extensor hallucis brevis) extend the toes. The muscles on the plantar (sole) side of the foot (flexor digitorum brevis, quadratus plantae, flexor hallucis brevis, flexor digiti minimi, abductor hallucis, abductor digiti minimi, plantar interosseous, lumbricales) are used to flex and spread the toes. Figures showing these muscles as well as a chart showing specific movements for each muscle are located at the end of the chapter (pages 138-140).

In normal daily activities, the muscles of the foot and lower leg are used more extensively than any other muscles in the body. Though the musculature of the lower leg is substantially smaller than that of the upper leg, it essentially supports the whole body and receives the heaviest load during walking or standing. As a result, many people have minor aches and pains in these muscles. Thus, at the end of the day people are ready to sit down and let these muscles rest. Stretching and strengthening these smaller muscle groups can alleviate some of the daily fatigue and pain. Stretching can also improve flexibility and stamina. These improvements enable the muscle groups to work harder and longer throughout the day.

Soreness, tightness, cramping, restlessness, and weakness in the arch of the foot and calf muscles are common complaints among people. These problems often result from the continuous and heavy load put on the muscle. Chronic use of these muscles can also increase muscle tightness and soreness. Tightness then leads to conditions such as tendinitis and shinsplints; tendinitis of the Achilles tendon is quite common. Tendinitis is associated with overuse and tightness of the gastrocnemius and soleus muscles. Shinsplints are associated with inflammation of the frontal compartment of the lower-leg muscles—anterior tibialis and, in some cases, soleus and flexor digitorum longus. These conditions can become excruciating if not treated in the early stages. A variety of stretching and strengthening exercises in those muscle groups will, in most cases, improve these conditions (lessen the severity) and help prevent future episodes from occurring. People often have delayed-onset muscle soreness, or DOMS, after participating in unusual or unfamiliar activities. Calf muscles tend to be affected by delayed-onset muscle soreness more often than any other muscle group in the body. Light stretching exercises help to improve this condition and relieve some of the pain associated with it.

All of the instructions and figures in this chapter are given for the right side of the body. Similar but opposite procedures would be used for the left side of the body.

Seated Toe Extensor Stretch

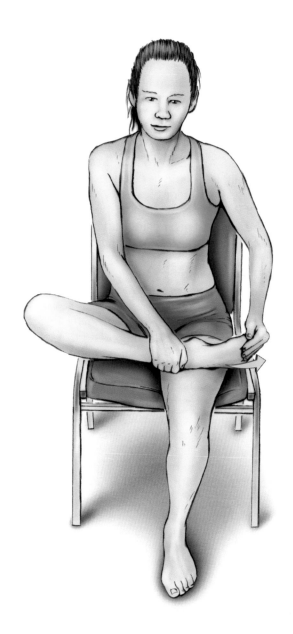

Technique

While sitting on a chair with the left foot on the floor, raise the right ankle and place it on top of the left knee.

While bracing the right ankle with the right hand, place the fingers of the left hand on the tops of the right toes.

Pull the tips of the toes toward the sole of the foot.

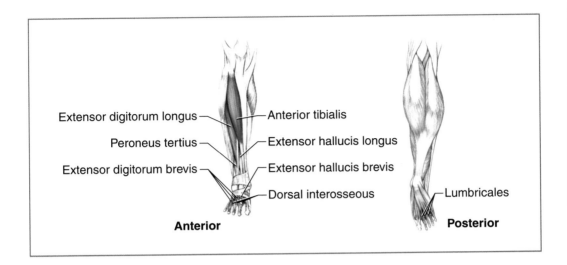

Extensor digitorum longus — Anterior tibialis
Peroneus tertius — Extensor hallucis longus
Extensor digitorum brevis — Extensor hallucis brevis
— Dorsal interosseous
— Lumbricales

Anterior   **Posterior**

Muscles Stretched

Most-stretched muscles: Right extensor digitorum longus, right extensor digi-torum brevis, right extensor hallucis longus, right extensor hallucis brevis, right anterior tibialis.

Lesser-stretched muscles: Right peroneus tertius, right dorsal interosseous, right lumbricales.

Commentary

Hold the ankle firmly in order to keep it and the foot stable. You will feel the stretch on the top of the foot area (dorsal side). If grasping and pulling on the tips of the toes cause too much pain, apply the pressure at the ball of the foot.

Seated Toe Extensor and Foot Everter Stretch

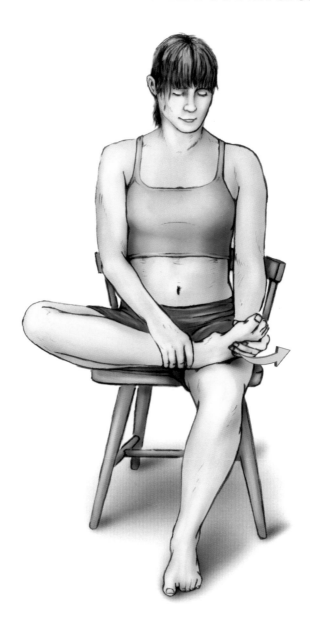

Technique

While sitting on a chair with the left foot on the floor, raise the right ankle and place it on top of the left knee.

While bracing the right ankle with the right hand, place the thumb of the left hand along the ball of the right foot and place the fingers of the left hand across the top of the foot with the fingers perpendicular to the toes.

Use the left hand to pull (or twist) the sole of the foot upward. At the same time, bend the toes toward the sole of the foot.

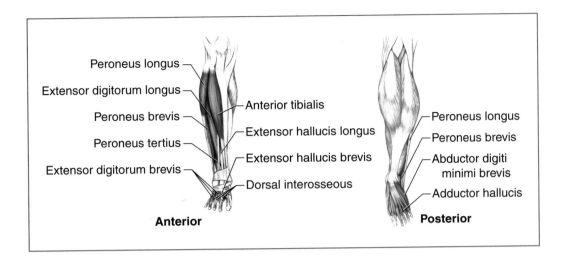

Anterior   **Posterior**

Muscles Stretched

Most-stretched muscles: Right extensor digitorum longus, right extensor digitorum brevis, right extensor hallucis longus, right extensor hallucis brevis, right dorsal interosseous, right abductor digiti minimi brevis, right adductor hallucis, right peroneus longus, right peroneus brevis, right peroneus tertius.

Lesser-stretched muscle: Right anterior tibialis.

Commentary

Make sure to stabilize the foot and ankle with a firm hold. Grasping the ends of the toes and pulling them upward (while keeping the toes in the flexed position) can produce a more effective stretch. You will feel the stretch on the lateral side of the foot (little toe side) and ankle area—abductor digiti minimi, extensor digitorum brevis, and extensor hallucis brevis muscles.

Seated Toe Extensor and Foot Inverter Stretch

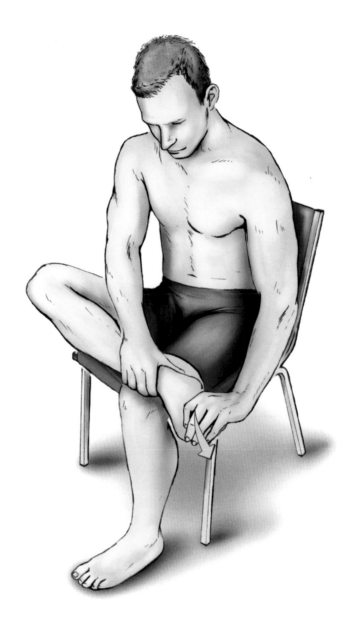

Technique

While sitting on a chair with left foot on the floor, raise the right ankle and place it on top of the left knee.

While bracing the right ankle with the right hand, place the thumb of the left hand along the ball of the right foot and the fingers of the left hand across the top of the foot with the fingers perpendicular to the toes.

Use the left hand to push (or twist) the sole of the foot down toward the floor. At the same time, bend the toes toward the sole of the foot.

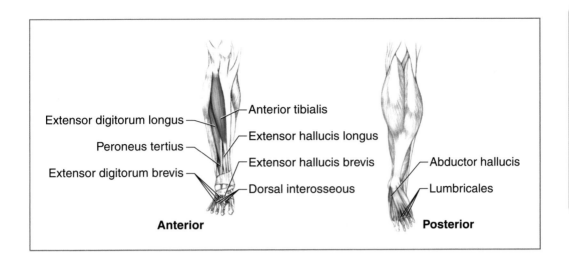

Anterior
- Extensor digitorum longus
- Peroneus tertius
- Extensor digitorum brevis
- Anterior tibialis
- Extensor hallucis longus
- Extensor hallucis brevis
- Dorsal interosseous

Posterior
- Abductor hallucis
- Lumbricales

Muscles Stretched

Most-stretched muscles: Right abductor hallucis, right extensor hallucis longus, right extensor hallucis brevis, right anterior tibialis.

Lesser-stretched muscles: Right extensor digitorum longus, right extensor digitorum brevis, right peroneus tertius, right lumbricales, right dorsal interosseous.

Commentary

Make sure to stabilize the foot and ankle with a firm hold. Grasping the ends of the toes and pressing them firmly downward can produce a greater stretch. You will feel the stretch on the medial side of the foot (big toe side).

Seated Toe Flexor Stretch

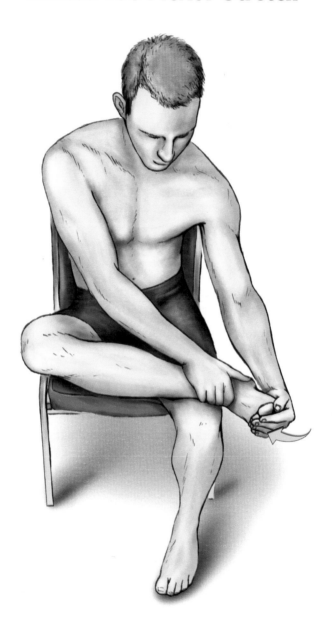

Technique

While sitting on a chair with the left foot on the floor, raise the right ankle and place it on top of the left knee.

Brace the right ankle with the right hand, and place the fingers of the left hand along the bottoms of the toes of the right foot with the fingers pointing in the same direction as the toes.

Use the fingers of the left hand to push the toes of the right foot toward the right knee.

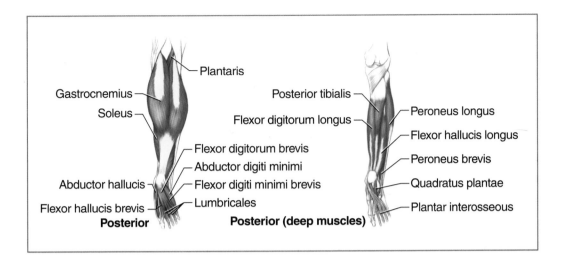

Muscles Stretched

Most-stretched muscles: Right flexor digitorum brevis, right quadratus plantae, right flexor digiti minimi brevis, right flexor hallucis brevis, right lumbricales, right plantar interosseous, right abductor hallucis, right abductor digiti minimi.

Lesser-stretched muscles: Right flexor digitorum longus, right flexor hallucis longus, right posterior tibialis, right peroneus longus, right peroneus brevis, right plantaris, right soleus, right gastrocnemius.

Commentary

Make sure to stabilize the foot and ankle with a firm hold. Pushing hard on the very ends of the toes with the left palm will provide a much greater stretch. You will feel the stretch on the sole (plantar side) of the foot.

Seated Toe Flexor and Foot Everter Stretch

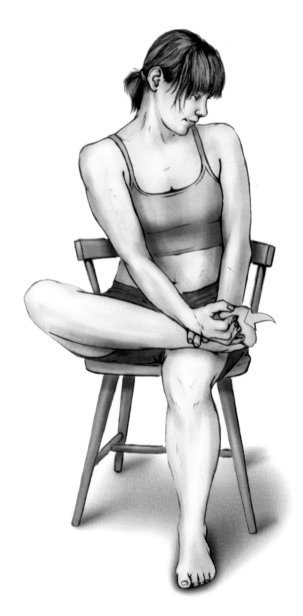

Technique

While sitting on a chair with the left foot on the floor, raise the right ankle and place it on top of the left knee.

Brace the right ankle with the left hand and place the fingers of the right hand perpendicular across the bottoms of the toes. Also place the pad of the right thumb on the ball of the right big toe.

Use the right hand to pull (or twist) the sole of the foot upward. At the same time, use the fingers of the right hand to pull the toes of the right foot up toward the top of the foot.

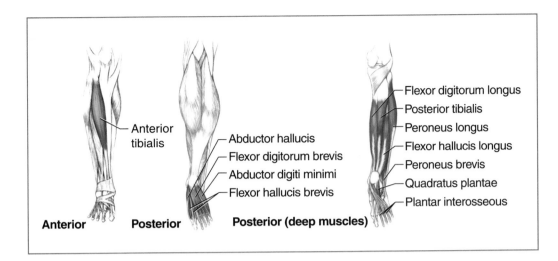

Anterior tibialis

Anterior

Abductor hallucis
Flexor digitorum brevis
Abductor digiti minimi
Flexor hallucis brevis

Posterior

Flexor digitorum longus
Posterior tibialis
Peroneus longus
Flexor hallucis longus
Peroneus brevis
Quadratus plantae
Plantar interosseous

Posterior (deep muscles)

Muscles Stretched

Most-stretched muscles: Right flexor digitorum brevis, right flexor hallucis brevis, right quadratus plantae, right abductor digiti minimi, right peroneus longus, right peroneus brevis, right plantar interosseous.

Lesser-stretched muscles: Right anterior tibialis, right flexor hallucis longus, right flexor digitorum longus, right posterior tibialis, right abductor hallucis.

Commentary

Make sure to stabilize the foot and ankle with a firm hold. If you grasp the very ends of the toes and pull harder, then you will be able to stretch these muscles even farther. You will feel the stretch on the sole (plantar side) of the foot.

Seated Toe Flexor and Foot Inverter Stretch

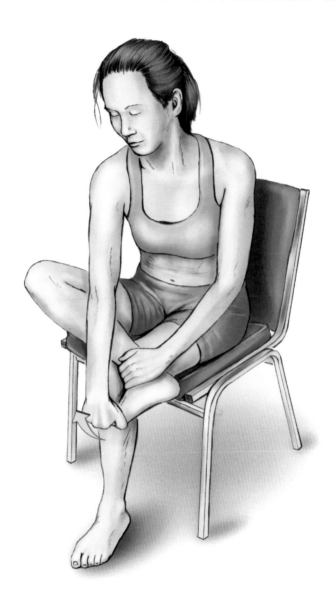

Technique

While sitting on a chair with the left foot on the floor, raise the right ankle and place it on top of the left knee.

Brace the right ankle with the left hand and place the fingers of the right hand perpendicular across the bottoms of the toes. Also place the pad of the right thumb on the ball of the right big toe.

Use the fingers of the right hand to pull the toes of the right foot up toward the top of the foot. At the same time, use the right thumb to push the sole of the right foot down toward the floor.

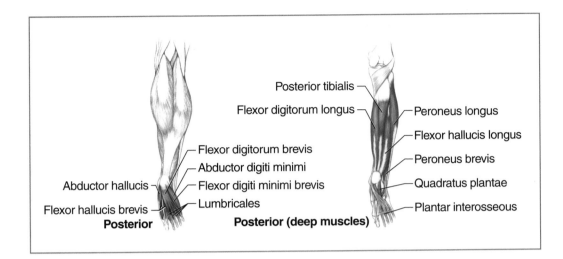

Posterior tibialis

Flexor digitorum longus

Peroneus longus

Flexor hallucis longus

Peroneus brevis

Flexor digitorum brevis

Abductor digiti minimi

Abductor hallucis

Flexor digiti minimi brevis

Quadratus plantae

Flexor hallucis brevis

Lumbricales

Plantar interosseous

Posterior

Posterior (deep muscles)

Muscles Stretched

Most-stretched muscles: Right flexor digitorum brevis, right quadratus plantae, right flexor digiti minimi brevis, right flexor hallucis brevis, right lumbricales, right plantar interosseous, right abductor hallucis.

Lesser-stretched muscles: Right peroneus longus, right peroneus brevis, right abductor digiti minimi, right flexor digitorum longus, right flexor hallucis longus, right posterior tibialis.

Commentary

Make sure to stabilize the foot and ankle with a firm hold. If you grasp the very ends of the toes and pull harder, then you will be able to stretch these muscles even farther. You will feel the stretch on the sole (plantar side) of the foot—the flexor digitorum brevis, flexor hallucis brevis, flexor digiti minimi brevis, and quadratus plantae muscles.

Standing Toe Extensor Stretch

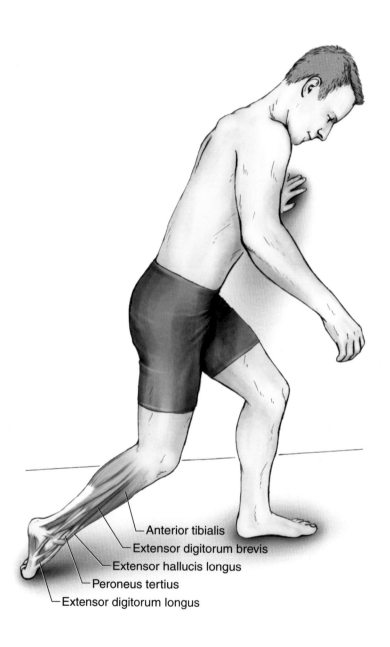

Anterior tibialis
Extensor digitorum brevis
Extensor hallucis longus
Peroneus tertius
Extensor digitorum longus

Technique

Stand upright and brace against a wall or an object for balance.

Point the right foot backward away from the body, dorsal (top) side of the toes down against the floor.

While keeping the dorsal side of the toes pressed against the floor, lean your weight onto the right leg and press the bottom of the heel down toward the floor.

Muscles Stretched

Most-stretched muscles: Right extensor digitorum brevis, right extensor hallucis brevis, right anterior tibialis, right peroneus tertius.

Lesser-stretched muscles: Right extensor hallucis longus, right extensor digitorum longus, right dorsal interosseous.

Commentary

It is more comfortable to perform this stretch on a carpet or other soft surface. Be sure not to drag the foot that is pressed to the floor. Moving the heel medially or laterally will place greater stretch on either the dorsal medial or dorsal lateral parts of the foot.

Standing Toe Flexor Stretch

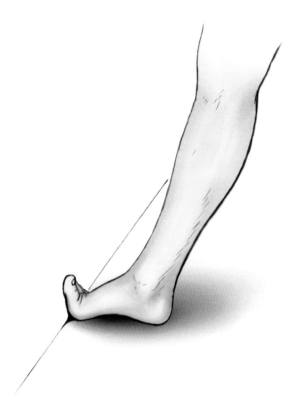

Technique

Stand upright while facing the wall, 1 to 2 feet (30 to 61 cm) away.

Keeping the heel of the foot on the floor, press the bottoms of the toes of the right foot up against the wall. The ball of the foot should be more than half an inch (more than 2 cm) above the floor.

Lean forward and slide the ball of the foot slowly down, keeping the toes pressed against the wall.

Muscles Stretched

Most-stretched muscles: Right flexor digitorum brevis, right quadratus plantae, right flexor digiti minimi brevis, right flexor hallucis brevis, right lumbricales, right plantar interosseous, right abductor hallucis, right abductor digiti minimi.

Lesser-stretched muscles: Right flexor digitorum longus, right flexor hallucis longus, right posterior tibialis.

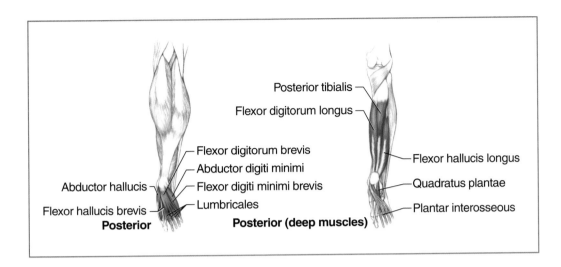

Posterior tibialis

Flexor digitorum longus

Flexor digitorum brevis

Abductor digiti minimi

Flexor digiti minimi brevis

Abductor hallucis

Lumbricales

Flexor hallucis brevis

Posterior

Flexor hallucis longus

Quadratus plantae

Plantar interosseous

Posterior (deep muscles)

Commentary

Make sure that the ball of the foot is parallel to the floor. This ensures that all of the toes are stretched equally. Also, slide the ball of the foot down slowly; otherwise, overstretching could happen. Bending the right knee slightly and moving the knee forward toward the wall will incorporate the calf muscles in the stretch.

Single Plantar Flexor Stretch

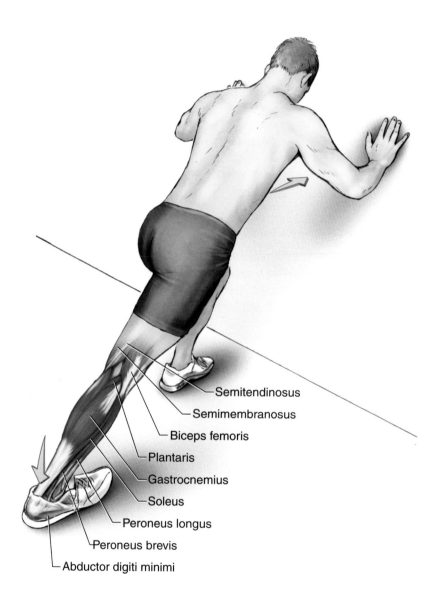

Semitendinosus

Semimembranosus

Biceps femoris

Plantaris

Gastrocnemius

Soleus

Peroneus longus

Peroneus brevis

Abductor digiti minimi

Technique

Stand facing a wall 2 feet (61 cm) away.

Brace your hands against the wall.

Keeping the left foot in place, place the right foot 1 to 2 feet (30 to 61 cm) behind the left foot. The left foot is 1 to 2 feet away and the right foot is 2 to 4 feet (61 to 122 cm) away from the wall.

Keeping the right heel on the floor, lean your chest toward the wall. You can bend the left knee slightly to facilitate moving the chest up against the wall.

Muscles Stretched

Most-stretched muscles: Right gastrocnemius, right soleus, right plantaris, right popliteus, right flexor digitorum longus, right flexor hallucis longus, right posterior tibialis.

Lesser-stretched muscles: Right peroneus longus, right peroneus brevis, right flexor digitorum brevis, right quadratus plantae, right flexor digiti minimi brevis, right flexor hallucis brevis, right abductor digiti minimi, right abductor hallucis, right popliteus, right semitendinosus, right semimembranosus, right biceps femoris.

Commentary

As the chest gets closer to the wall, bending the knee slightly will realign the tibia and increase the distance between the muscle attachment points. This will increase the stretch on the posterior tibialis, flexor hallucis longus, and flexor digitorum longus muscles while at the same time reducing the stretch on the hamstring muscles.

Double Plantar Flexor Stretch

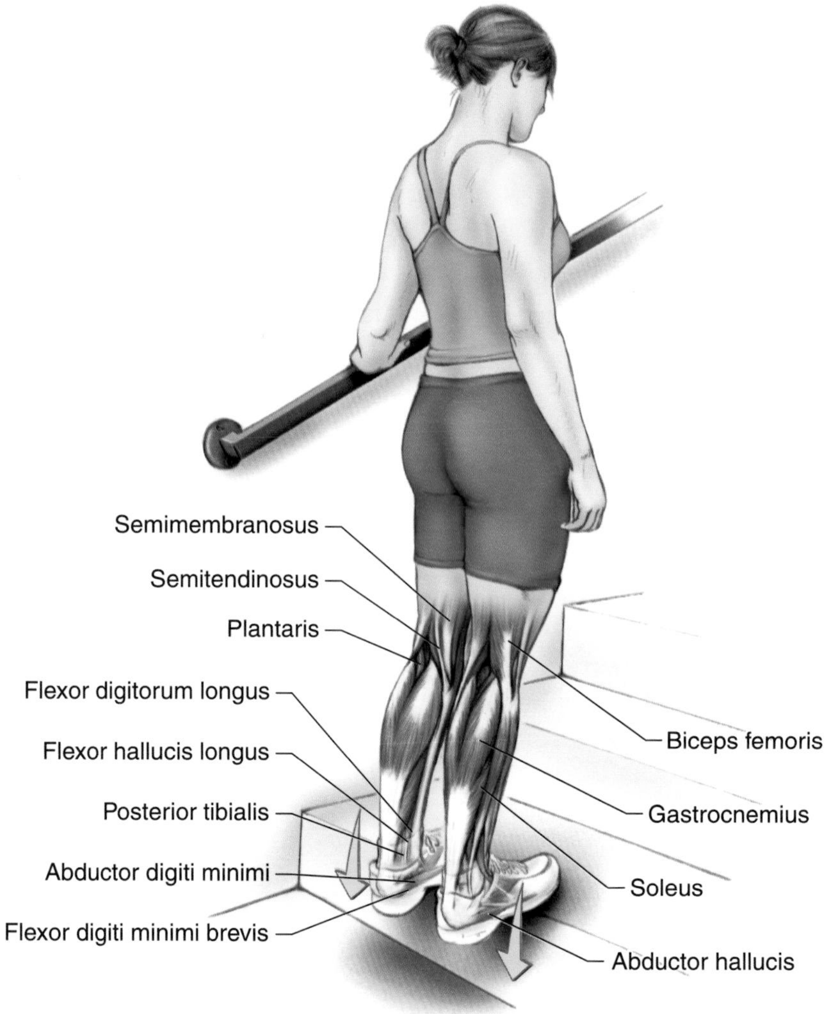
Semimembranosus
Semitendinosus
Plantaris
Flexor digitorum longus
Flexor hallucis longus
Posterior tibialis
Abductor digiti minimi
Flexor digiti minimi brevis
Biceps femoris
Gastrocnemius
Soleus
Abductor hallucis

Technique

Stand upright on the edge of a stair or beam, with both heels unsupported out past the edge.

Keep the right and left knees straight, and hold on to a support with at least one hand.

Lower both heels down as far as possible.

Muscles Stretched

Most-stretched muscles: Gastrocnemius, soleus, plantaris, popliteus, flexor digitorum longus, flexor digitorum brevis, flexor hallucis longus, flexor hallucis brevis, posterior tibialis, quadratus plantae, flexor digiti minimi brevis, abductor digiti minimi, abductor hallucis.

Lesser-stretched muscles: Semitendinosus, semimembranosus, biceps femoris.

Commentary

It is more comfortable to do this stretch while wearing shoes. Always support the body—an unsupported body could cause the muscles to contract and not stretch. You will increase the extent of the stretch if you work one leg at a time. After the heels reach their lowest point, you can apply more stretch by bending the knees slightly. This will stretch the posterior tibialis, flexor hallucis longus, and flexor digitorum longus muscles; at the same time it will reduce the stretch on the hamstring muscles. Placing the ball of the foot on the edge of the stairs or beam will increase the stretch on the origin (top part) of these muscle groups. Placing the midsection of the foot on the edge of the stairs or beam increases the stretch on the lower portion of these muscles.

Plantar Flexor and Foot Everter Stretch

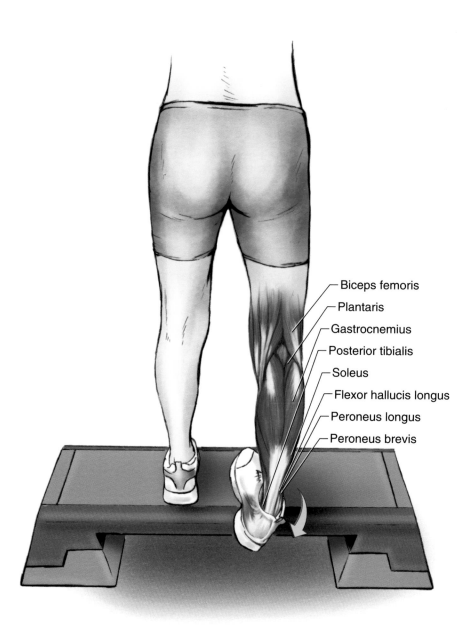

Biceps femoris

Plantaris

Gastrocnemius

Posterior tibialis

Soleus

Flexor hallucis longus

Peroneus longus

Peroneus brevis

134

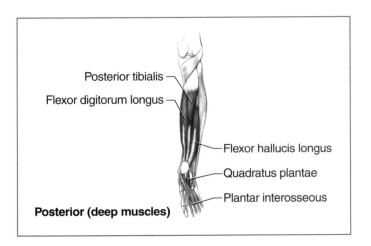

Posterior tibialis

Flexor digitorum longus

Flexor hallucis longus

Quadratus plantae

Plantar interosseous

Posterior (deep muscles)

Technique

Stand upright on the edge of a stair or beam, with the midsection of the right foot on the edge.

Place the foot in an inverted position (stand on the lateral [outer] side of the foot).

Keep the right knee straight and the left knee slightly bent.

Hold on to a support with at least one hand.

Keeping the foot inverted, lower the right heel as far as possible.

Muscles Stretched

Most-stretched muscles: Right peroneus longus, right peroneus brevis, right peroneus tertius, right abductor digiti minimi, lateral side of right soleus and right gastrocnemius, right flexor hallucis longus, right posterior tibialis.

Lesser-stretched muscles: Right popliteus, right plantaris, medial head of right gastrocnemius, right biceps femoris, right flexor digitorum brevis, right quadratus plantae, right flexor digiti minimi brevis, right flexor hallucis brevis.

Commentary

It is more comfortable to do this stretch while wearing shoes. This is an excellent stretch for the peroneus longus and brevis and the abductor digiti minimi muscles, which are located at the lateral (outer) side of the lower leg and the foot. Be extra careful when placing the foot in an inverted position, and make sure to progress slowly through this stretching exercise. After the right heel reaches the floor or the lowest point, you can increase the stretch by bending the right knee slightly. This removes any stretch on hamstring muscles, but it stretches the calf muscles further.

Plantar Flexor and Foot Inverter Stretch

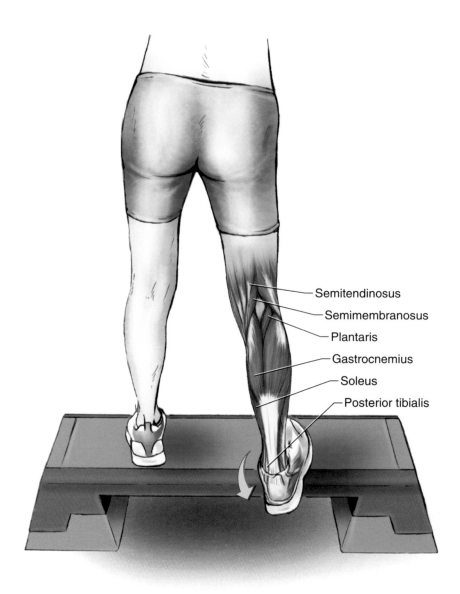

Semitendinosus
Semimembranosus
Plantaris
Gastrocnemius
Soleus
Posterior tibialis

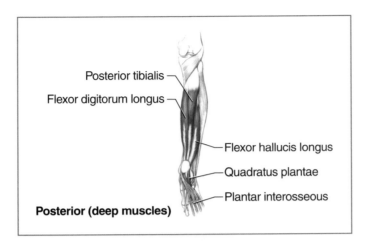

Posterior tibialis

Flexor digitorum longus

Flexor hallucis longus

Quadratus plantae

Plantar interosseous

Posterior (deep muscles)

Technique

Stand upright on the edge of a stair or beam, with the midsection of the right foot on the edge.

Place the foot in an everted position (stand on the medial [inner] side of the foot).

Bend the right knee slightly toward the midsection of the body (inside direction), with the left knee slightly bent.

Hold on to a support with at least one hand.

While keeping the foot everted, lower the right heel as far as possible.

Muscles Stretched

Most-stretched muscles: Right flexor digitorum longus, right abductor hallucis, medial side of right soleus, right posterior tibialis, right plantaris.

Lesser-stretched muscles: Right flexor digitorum brevis, right quadratus plantae, right flexor hallucis brevis, right flexor digiti minimi brevis, right medial gastrocnemius, right semitendinosus, right semimembranosus.

Commentary

It is more comfortable to do this stretch while wearing shoes. This is an excellent stretch for the flexor digitorum longus, medial soleus, and abductor hallucis muscles, which are located at the medial side of the lower leg and foot. Take extra care when placing the foot in an everted position, and make sure to progress slowly through this stretching position. After the right heel reaches the floor or the lowest point, bending the right knee slightly can increase the stretch. This reduces the stretch on hamstring muscles, but it increases the stretch on the calf muscles.

Foot and Calf Muscle Movements

The stretches in this chapter are excellent overall stretches; however, not all of these stretches may be completely suited to each person's needs. The muscles involved in the various calf, ankle, and foot movements appear in the following table. To stretch specific muscles, the stretch must involve one or more movements in the opposite direction of the desired muscle's movements. For example, if you want to stretch the left flexor digitorum longus, you could perform a movement that involves dorsiflexion and eversion of the left ankle and toe extension of the left foot. When a muscle has a high level of stiffness, you should use fewer simultaneous opposite movements (for example, to stretch a very tight flexor digitorum longus, you could start by doing only toe extension). As a muscle becomes loose, you can incorporate more simultaneous opposite movements.

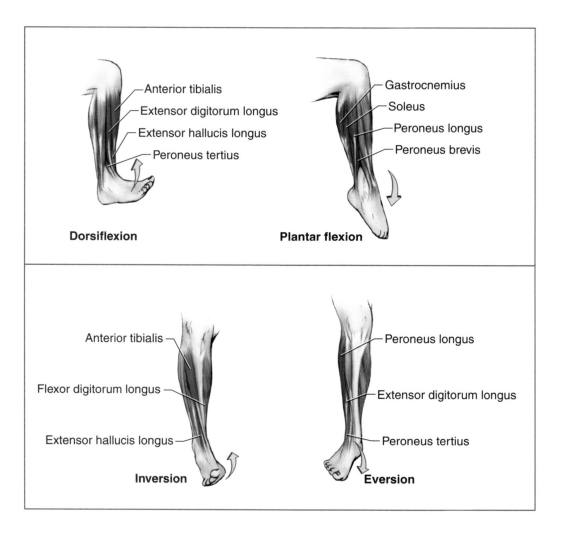

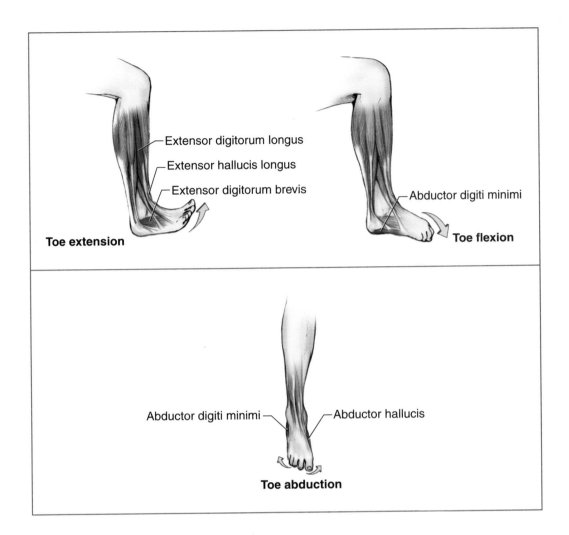

Extensor digitorum longus

Extensor hallucis longus

Extensor digitorum brevis

Toe extension

Abductor digiti minimi

Toe flexion

Abductor digiti minimi

Abductor hallucis

Toe abduction

LOWER LEG

Muscle	Dorsi-flexion	Plantar flexion	Foot inversion	Foot eversion	Toe extension	Toe flexion
Anterior tibialis	✔		✔			
Extensor digitorum longus	✔			✔	✔	
Extensor hallucis longus	✔		✔		✔	
Peroneus tertius	✔			✔		
Peroneus longus		✔		✔		
Peroneus brevis		✔		✔		
Gastrocnemius		✔				
Soleus		✔				
Plantaris		✔				
Posterior tibialis		✔	✔			
Flexor digitorum longus		✔	✔			✔
Flexor hallucis longus		✔	✔			✔

FOOT

Muscle	Toe extension	Toe flexion	Toe abduction
Flexor digitorum brevis		✔	
Quadratus plantae		✔	
Flexor digiti minimi brevis		✔	
Abductor hallucis		✔	✔
Abductor digiti minimi		✔	✔
Adductor hallucis		✔	
Flexor hallucis brevis		✔	
Extensor digitorum brevis	✔		
Extensor hallucis brevis	✔		
Lumbricales	✔	✔	
Plantar interosseus		✔	
Dorsal interosseus	✔		

STRETCH INDEX

ABOUT THE AUTHORS

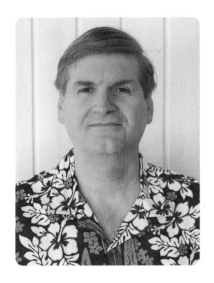

Arnold G. Nelson, PhD, is an associate professor in the department of kinesiology at Louisiana State University. A leading researcher on flexibility, he is considered one of the top authorities on how stretching affects muscle performance. Nelson is a fellow of the American College of Sports Medicine and earned his PhD in muscle physiology from the University of Texas at Austin. He resides in Baton Rouge, Louisiana, with his wife, Kathy.

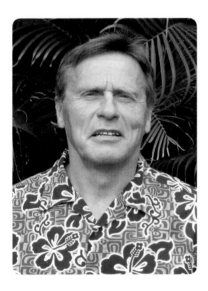

Jouko Kokkonen, PhD, is a professor in exercise science at Brigham Young University in Hawaii. For more than 20 years, he has taught anatomy, kinesiology, exercise physiology, and athletic conditioning, and for 35 years he has coached track and field. Kokkonen's research has revolved around the acute and chronic effects of stretching. He earned his PhD in exercise physiology from Brigham Young and now resides in Laie, Hawaii, with his wife, Ruthanne.

ABOUT THE ILLUSTRATOR

Jason M. McAlexander, MFA, founded Quail Ridge Studios in 2004, where he specializes in scientific and medical illustrations in both traditional and digital media. Previously, he served as art director and chief illustrator for a multinational publishing company based in Portland, Oregon. McAlexander received his bachelor's degree in biological and premedical illustration from Iowa State University and went on to receive his master of fine arts degree in medical and biological illustration from the University of Michigan.

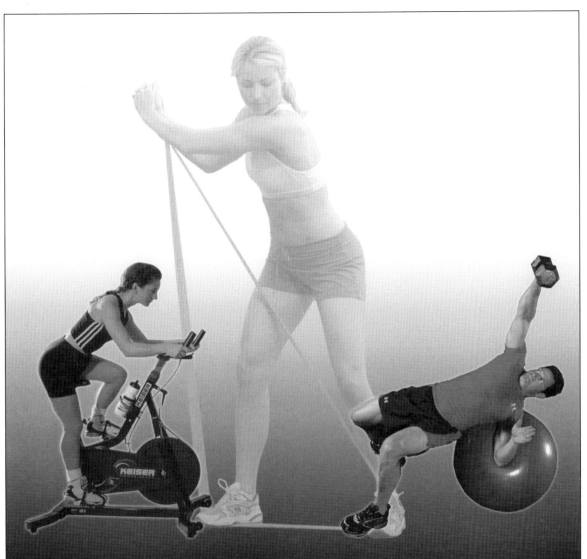

You'll find other outstanding fitness resources at

http://fitness.humankinetics.com

In the U.S. call 1-800-747-4457

Australia 08 8372 0999 • Canada 1-800-465-7301
Europe +44 (0) 113 255 5665 • New Zealand 0064 9 448 1207

HUMAN KINETICS
The Premier Publisher for Sports & Fitness
P.O. Box 5076 • Champaign, IL 61825-5076 USA